SLIMMING DOWN

SLIMMING DOWN
BY ED McMAHON

GROSSET & DUNLAP
A National General Company
Publishers   New York

CONTENTS

1.
I Was Overweight at Birth

It's all my grandmother's fault. She was Katie Fitzgerald, a lovely lady. She bolted from the Boston Fitzgerald clan and married this renegade plumber named Joe McMahon. They had a happy life together, at least as far as I could tell.

She bore all of Joe's progeny, nine of whom made it to the first grade. As the family grew, one of Katie's older lads, Ed, married and fathered a son named Edward. He was, according to reliable reports, fat, happy, smiling, cute and winsome. So much so, that Katie took me to her bosom and board and that's how it all began.

All our meals were served by Grandma Katie. They were substantial enough to be chosen by captured spies as their last meal.

Creamed potatoes for breakfast, pork chops, pan-fried cabbage from the night before, apples and cheese and that tiny little home-made loaf of bread prepared just for little Edward. Breakfast sometimes lasted so long there was al-

3

most no time to push our chairs back from the table to get up and brush our teeth, before it was lunch time. That meant more potatoes, a choice meat and a wide assortment of cakes, pies and other goodies.

Naturally there were potatoes at every meal, a carry-over from the harsh times in Ireland brought about by the potato famine. And since potatoes are one of the biggest sources of carbohydrates—the dieter's worst enemy—you can see I was off to a bad start as far as attaining a tapered figure was concerned. But we ate, and we ate plenty. And we loved every bit of it.

Because people were starving in China and India and Ethiopia, we had to eat every bit on our plates. No one knew why. No one except Katie Fitzgerald and she wasn't telling. At least she never told me. But she stood there until we cleaned our plates. I vaguely recall her telling me —even then—to lick my platter clean because people were starving in Pakistan. To the best of my knowledge there wasn't even a Pakistan in existence at the time, but Katie, in a remarkable bit of prophetic divination, had me eating for the future hungry of the world. And so I ate. People were starving someplace, but we were full to bursting at Katie's table.

And by the way, she made the greatest blueberry pie in all the world. Escoffier would have cried if he had tasted her pie. The Mystery Chef would have renounced his culinary vows. The Galloping Gourmet—well, you get the idea. Great blueberry pie!

So, with no rancor or ill-will, I must state that it was all Katie Fitzgerald's fault. For want of a better place to begin, let's begin there.

I was overweight at birth. Officially I was tabbed at the weigh-in as 9 pounds, 14 ounces, approximately one-third above the national average, a fractional disproportion I've been fighting to stay under much of my life.

My school years just represented a change of locale for my epicurean histrionics. My school lunches, presided over chiefly by Grandma Katie, might best be described as a moveable feast. My lunchbox, when properly packed, contained six sandwiches and a quart of milk. Packing my lunchbox was tantamount to packing another kid's suitcase for a two-week stay at camp.

This bountiful collection of edibles lasted until about 10 A.M., when the pangs of hunger would gnaw at my innards, setting me to prowl about the schoolyard, panther-like, in the hope of getting a stray macaroon or pumpernickel crust from a friendly classmate.

The years passed by quickly and I grew taller and a little wider. Medical men today might have referred to me as an adipescent adolescent. Everything I ate seemed to go right to my waist and hips and stay there. Naturally I was still consuming the potatoes, bread and sweets that had made me happy, jolly and husky during my formative years.

I don't recall the exact year, but I suddenly shot up in height and thinned down considerably. And for one glorious segment of my existence I was known as "Skinny." Excuse me for a moment while I dwell on that — "Skinny" McMahon. What can I say? That's sheer poetry.

But that delightful epoch soon faded into oblivion, taking my short-lived nickname with it. I reverted to my original form and noted with growing dismay that the fat was coming back to my body. It was the real start of my life-long battle against the adipose tissue seeking a permanent home on my frame.

One comforting factor is that I'm not alone in my fight against fat. According to a recent survey, more than sixty million Americans right now are searching to find the right diet to suit their own particular needs and desires. More than sixty million! And I'm one of them.

Studies show that diet-conscious Americans lose, and then regain, 250 million pounds a year. Right now Americans are toting around a billion surplus pounds on their bodies. If you don't believe it, just look around.

Americans concerned about their weight go on an average of one-and-a-quarter diets a year. But since most diets present such a strict regimen with overpowering lists of "no-no's," the majority of the would-be slimmers fall right off the dieting wagon. It's difficult to obey a diet that demands you eliminate *everything* you crave and are used to. I think this is why I, and millions of others, have had so much trouble in the past.

Now I'm no voluptuary. I'm not a disciple of Epicurus who pushed the good life back in 3000 B.C. I'm just an average, hard-working human who's trying to do a good job, make a buck and keep reasonably slim, trim and healthy. And so I have dieted. To paraphrase Mark Twain's famous remark about giving up smoking, I might say, "giving up things you like to eat and drink is easy. I've done it many times." Believe me, my efforts to achieve a certain sleekness have taken me along many weird dietary trails.

I've tried the Apple Diet, the Grape Diet, the North Pole Slenderizing Plan, several "magic formula" diets, the Drinking Man's Diet (at the urging of my friends), the 8-Day Diet (completed in five days) and many others whose names escape me right now. Oh, I'm not saying I didn't lose weight. I did. For a while. But it came back.

Medical men today agree that obesity problems are psychological rather than abdominal. That is, the trouble is rooted in the mind instead of the stomach. To be successful, a diet must satisfy your belly's craving for bulk, but more important, it must soothe you mentally and emotionally, filling your intangible need that goes back to your childhood (ah there, Grandma Katie) and revolves around your day-to-day existence. And let me say, your job does influence your ability to adhere to a diet.

I'm not trying to cop out, but my job offers unique opportunities to indulge myself gastronomically, to partake fully of the joyous ambrosia and nectar of the gods. Fate has a way of throwing emotional obstacles in your path as you go through life; her way of checking your inner strength.

Believe me, when you're trying to lose weight and you have lunch with someone like Johnny Carson—*that's* an obstacle. We walk into a restaurant together and before I get my bib in place, Johnny's finished three breadsticks and is starting on his fourth. I sit there, fumbling with the silverware, deliberately keeping my hands occupied so I won't grab a breadstick or two as a warm-up for the meal. He reaches for another one and I tremble with hunger and a fierce desire to take a bite that will send my carbohydrate count for the day soaring into the "fatso" level So I desist—that time. What the next outing with Johnny will bring, and how I will react, I never know But I think I have the answer.

I don't have a name for it and I don't like to call it a diet, because it's not really that. For purposes of identification, let's call it the Ed McMahon Slimming System. True, breadsticks aren't favored, but the system does allow me to have my martinis, eat my fill of steaks, fish and cheese. And yes, it even permits me a midnight snack when I'm home watching my favorite late night talk show on TV along with a bottle of Budweiser.

I want to give credit where credit is due. As I mentioned, I tried dozens of diets to no avail until I stumbled across (sorry, make that *came* across) a fine book called *Martinis & Whipped Cream* by Sidney Petrie and Robert B. Stone. It's in a Paperback Library edition and it opened my eyes to a new way of getting rid of fat for good. Naturally, being an irrepressible improviser, I added a few variations of my own.

Our world is filled with tension, disruptions of schedule and a frenzied pace of pressures that can destroy the determined efforts of even the most conscientious dieter.

Take flying. I do a lot of flying and each trip is a test of willpower for me. You get a seat on the plane. You're early. Or maybe there's a delay. A pretty girl in uniform puts a strange looking potato with scalloped edges in front of you. When I'm in top form on my home ground this potato presents no problem at all. But seated on a plane, waiting, waiting—that's the time this skimpy spud in front of me begins to look like the juiciest T-bone steak in town. More temptations to weaken one.

Perhaps you commute to work each day. I've done that, too. Commuting is great for conviviality, meeting friends, doing a little public relations work or discussing business. And isn't all of this a bit easier if done over a few libations? Most libations aren't going to put weight on you (one of the features of my plan), but you soon find yourself reaching for the strategically placed peanuts, chips, nuts and other assorted goodies designed to turn you jowly.

Drinking men will profit by my plan, too. How could a drinking man take orders from a diet that prevents him from indulging now and then? Impossible. My plan doesn't present any such restrictions. You want that second martini? Fine. Third? Sure. It's all in what you do later that counts and I'll go into that in a subsequent chapter.

If you're a housewife who has gone up and down the scales regularly trying diets that work for a time and then fail to hold you, I can help. Sure, you find yourself cleaning the leavings of the children's morning cereals and the scraps from the evening meal. Yes, you're in the habit of making coffee and treating yourself to a pastry while watching your daytime serials. It's rough. But the system I use will satisfy your hunger pangs and get you back to that trimness that you (and your husband) were so proud of.

Newlyweds take heed. Many young grooms run to fat a few years after being spoiled by the little woman who wants to impress with her cooking skills. This book will offer some menus and advice on shopping that will keep the scales weighted in your favor.

Probably the biggest reason why you should stay slim is health. Hippocrates, the Greek medic once said, "Sudden death is more common in those who are naturally fat than in those who are lean." And let me say that a look at some actuarial charts tells you that the old boy knew what he was talking about.

Insurance companies tell us that a man in his thirties who is overweight by 25 per cent is reducing his life expectancy by as much as twelve years! That's a lot of great days and nights of fun to give up because you couldn't say no to some starchy foods. So why not embark on a new life-style that is geared toward your full quota of years filled with health, good-times and happiness?

There are no harsh deprivations to drive you up a wall. No rigid strictures to turn you into a grumbling, nervous neurotic. Nothing that demands you shut out the joyful vibrations of life.

I'm not saying it's ridiculously simple. There are some requirements.

You'll need common sense, a certain willpower which will enable you to press your nose against the window of life's candy store occasionally without going in, a desire to be streamlined and the ability to say no once in a while.

It's a battle, but we've got the weapons.

So we're in this together, ladies and gentlemen.

Now, if you'll excuse me, I have to go out and earn my daily bread. (One thin slice, please. Hold the butter.)

2.
The Breadstick
Conspiracy

My preparation for the "Tonight Show" begins at 4:30 P.M. with the appearance of the make-up man. He touches me up in his artful manner and I begin mulling over the line-up of guests appearing on the show. Although the show is seen from 11:30 P.M. to 1:00 A.M., the taping is done at 6 P.M.

I've already gone through the list of live commercials (as opposed to those already taped), and I check the rundown to see if I'll be working with Johnny on any comedy bits.

As I approach each show a sense of excitement starts to build. There's something about doing a show in front of a live audience that is exhilarating. I can be fighting fatigue, a head cold or a rebellious stomach, but when I stride out in front of the cameras and talk to the packed house all my difficulties fade away.

Our audiences come from all over the country. Many of them have waited ten months to get tickets (they're free) for the show. I follow the producer and our clotheshorse conductor, Doc Severinsen, out to greet the already happy crowd. I may open with a cheery, "How are you?" to the full house. If the response isn't overpowering (often audience members are a little hesitant to respond) I'll call out, "Now what kind of a response is that? I've waited all day to see you. Now let's hear it. How are you?"

That usually inspires an eardrum-threatening chorus and I go into my three or four-minute warm-up before introducing Johnny.

I'll occasionally warn the men in the audience that the cameras will be trained on the crowd in exactly one hour for the audience shot (which you see at 12:30 A.M.) and advise them that if they're with someone they shouldn't be with, well, it might be wise for them to slump down or leave right now so they won't be seen by the little woman back home.

Next I'll do a story or two dispelling those awful rumors started by Johnny's jokes about my drinking. By now the clock's hand is nearing the big moment when "Skinny," as I refer to him in the warm-up, strolls out from behind the curtain.

"How much time?" I ask.

"One," says the producer, meaning one minute.

"I'll take one," I reply, "very dry, with an olive."

The theme music starts and then I let go with, "And now, heeeerr's Johnny!" And another show is underway.

I've been doing the show with Johnny for more than nine years and I still get a thrill out of going out and facing the audience and participating in the sometimes wild, sometimes serious goings-on that the show has become famous for. Actually I've worked with Johnny for nearly fifteen years. He hired me after a five-minute interview for his previous show, "Who Do You Trust."

People say we hit it off so well together on stage it

looks as if we'd spent hours rehearsing. There's practically no rehearsal at all except for a brief moment or two going over the sketches we perform occasionally.

One reason it comes across so well is that Johnny and I have a good, natural give-and-take attitude. He's the boss, the star, the comic. I'm the announcer, second banana, the average guy gainfully employed. I've been told that men feel they can relate to me because I'm doing a day-to-day job just as they are. And when I'm able to give the boss an occasional zinger, there's empathy between myself and millions of men out there who'd like to do the same thing.

There are lots of bosses in the world who use their power unwisely. You know the type. They'll take advantage of their position to put down an employee. Maybe it's about his baldness or toothiness, something visual that becomes an easy target for remarks. Usually, these jibes are heard only by a few people and that's that. Now those of you who see the show know that Johnny likes to unload a few barbs at me about my size and weight. And each insult is heard by countless millions.

This is the type of material Johnny will hit me with during one of his monologues.

"Ed did a wonderful act of charity recently. During a severe rainstorm he let a family of midgets huddle under his belly."

Or, "The airline gives garment bags to the entire staff for our trip to California—even Ed. His is a little unusual. He has the only garment bag roomy enough to sleep six."

Or, "You all know Ed McMahon—the Bluebird of Flabbiness."

Now I ask you, is that any way to treat a faithful, trusted employee who's labored in the vineyards of commercial TV with one man almost fifteen years?

But it's all in fun, it helps the show, I'm getting used to it and besides . . . he *is* the boss.

However, there is one particular area in our relationship that is really tough to take, particularly now that I'm on a diet. That area is eating in a restaurant with Johnny and being victimized by the dreaded Breadstick Conspiracy.

Now bread is one of the foods to be avoided on my diet, chiefly because it is rich in carbohydrates. Briefly, my reducing program—it's not really a diet as you will see—cuts down on carbohydrates which many doctors believe, and I am convinced, are the real culprits in depositing fatty tissues on your frame. We'll go into it in more detail later. Let's pick up at the restaurant.

It's a nice place on Manhattan's East Side. The floors are clean, the waiters polite and the tablecloths are spotless. However, placed before me is a mountain of breadsticks in all shapes and sizes—long, round, gnarled, pumpernickel, French, Italian—piled into a wicker basket. I turn away my eyes. This is bad news. One small French roll has 100 calories (before buttering), and more important in my scheme of things, sixty-five of those calories are in carbohydrates. For convenience's sake, let's refer to them as carbo-cals.

Now you take four or five of those rolls and you've taken my recommended carbo-cal supply for the entire day! I pretend the breadsticks and rolls aren't there. I avert my eyes with great effort and begin noticing things about the room. Things like is that waitress smiling at me or snarling. That kind of speculation doesn't work for long because there in front of me, heeeerrr's Johnny hoisting a breadstick lathered with butter. This is no ordinary breadstick. This could be used for major league batting practice. He finishes the first breadstick, picks up another and the ensuing conversation goes this way:

"I think what we should do on this, Ed, is to (bites breadstick) go ahead as planned (chomp) and if he wants to change (chomp, chomp) well, we'll come up with (big bite) something (two bites) that's mutually satisfactory (bite, chomp, bite, chomp, chomp)."

He finishes the sentence, reaches for another breadstick, soaks it with butter and resumes. I die a little with each chomp. I've eaten with Johnny for a long time now. Fifteen years of eating breadsticks and he's still as skinny as a pipe cleaner.

I take some solace in the fact that he always has been abnormally thin. The story is that when he was a boy he was so thin the other kids used to scale him into the lake to see who could make him skip the most times across the water.

But then, as a boy, I was never overweight. I was tall and I ate an awful lot, but I wasn't considered fat.

Through my football years in high school (Lowell, Mass.) and college (Boston) I maintained a good weight for my height. But as you get older and your energy output drops, your food input should drop accordingly. That, friends, as those of you who've tried dieting before, is the hard part. Now having gotten this far in life, you might just feel you're entitled to a few of the goodies. And you are. But you must be wise in picking those goodies. I have developed my own plan to triumph over the insidious Breadstick Conspiracy.

When I no longer can ignore the bulging bread pile and find my right hand inching involuntarily toward the basket, I snap into action, summon a waiter and order a martini. After all, man does not live by bread alone. And look at it this way, a martini does have about 200 calories, granted, but it contains only one carbo-cal. Do you realize I could have *sixty-five* martinis to equal the carbo-cals of one French roll?

But martinis are not taboo on my program. You can have them in modest quantities. And I must say I am always modest about the quantities I have. After all, we're not ascetics or stoics put here to deprive ourselves of everything nice. It's just that in my case it's wiser (and more refreshing) to substitute a martini for that fattening, carbohydrate-loaded French roll.

"Waiter, bring me another, please." I'm about to substitute for two French rolls.

Johnny's not the only tempter I encounter along the road to my trim heaven. The Breadstick Conspiracy is universal in scope. It rears its calorie head at every luncheon meeting or banquet. I do a lot of speaking to different groups. Often it takes a lot of time for the others to get done talking so I can have my turn. You'd be surprised how two gentlemen in dark suits can stand up, open with, "I'll only say a few words," and kill the better part of an hour. So there I sit, staring at the crowd staring at me, smiling, nodding, unraveling. It's unnerving. What do I do? Right. Reach for the bread. Ah, there's the butter right near my elbow. How convenient. I dab some butter on my puffed-up roll and soon another day's dieting bites the dust.

I occasionally go to restaurant lunches with large groups of people from a company or advertising agency. That's another potential area of devastation. Now a martini is fine, and two are better. But to be perfectly frank, a diet of soft drink is best when you're trying to lose weight. The typical low-calorie soft drink contains only two calories per eight-ounce glass and no carbo-cals at all. After feeling a little guilty about falling away from my planned eating program over the weekend, I've been known to get the waiter's attention and shout, "Sixteen Tabs all around," or "Fresca for everyone. It's on me."

That sometimes works, but I must admit that I see a few quizzical glances being exchanged behind me. I'm sure it doesn't enhance my image as bon vivant or gourmet extraordinaire. Can you trust a man who gorges himself and everyone else on low-calorie soft drinks? It takes backbone to project that kind of an image, but that's the sort of raw courage that separates the men from the boys.

My working schedule is oft-times erratic. I travel a lot, work odd hours on a lot of things besides the "Tonight Show," and I frequently find myself ingesting my big meal just before bedtime. As you know, the worst time to eat heavily is just before you go to sleep. Your stomach is loaded and it stays loaded. Unless you're the world's most active sleepwalker you get no exercise at all, and that big meal you just ate hangs in there like a mass of reinforced concrete, except this concrete gurgles at you—just to make doubly sure that you stay awake to keep it company.

These late night eat-ins are further complicated if you're voracious, and a prime target for those ever-present seductive breadsticks that lie in wait, ready to ambush you again. Your willpower is being tested once more.

"Half a loaf is better than no bread," said John Heywood, back in the sixteenth century. And while it may be philosophically true, you can bet that was one philosopher who wasn't dieting. Half a loaf—of bread—could wipe me, and my weight-reducing plans, out.

By heredity or environment, or whatever happened during my formative years (all factors that strongly influence your eating patterns, psychologists agree), all I know is that I'm a sucker for breads. *Bread.* BREAD. BREAD! You name it, and I want it. French, Italian, Syrian, English buns, croissants, long loaves or round, Jewish rye or German pumpernickel. If you have that problem with bread, then you and I share the same mental anguish when confronted by the dough-laden Lorelei and its silent siren song luring us to our plumpish fate.

Now bread isn't the only diet destroyer. It just happens

to be one of my major weaknesses. Yours may be different. What I want to do in explaining my personal program and problems, is to first make you aware of the items you should avoid or cut back on. And bread is one of the biggies.

But let me reassure you by listing some of the foods which you can eat in goodly amounts—just so you won't think I'm pushing you into the yawning pit of starvation. You can regale yourself with steak, and ham, and bacon, and eggs, and cheeses, and fish, and pork, and turkey, and chicken, and mushrooms, and lettuce, and string beans, and spinach, and mayonnaise, and cauliflower, and onions, and melons, *and . . . and . . . and . . . .* That's just for openers, just to keep you thinking positively, happily while you're girding your mind to the business of losing weight.

All of these items are very low in carbo-cal content. And while we're on this joyous note, let me recommend another list which is only a bit higher in carbo-cals to add to your roster of helpful, filling foodstuffs. They're cold cuts and grapefruit, tomato juice and broccoli, carrots and dessert mixes. Now that's a wide range of delicacies that you can get your teeth into without worrying about adding another inch or so to that waistline. Don't feel that the shrinking man must torture himself into zombie-dom with a rigid no-taste diet.

The reasons people overeat are complex. They involve parental influences, frustration, unhappiness, desire to be loved. Certainly you're not going to have a successful diet if you burden your already overburdened psyche with more strict unyielding regulations.

As Dr. Philip White of the American Medical Association says, "A diet that does not take into consideration the psychological reasons why a person eats is almost certainly doomed to failure."

In other words, most of us derive considerable satisfaction from eating, and my diet takes this into account. That's why I think you'll be able to follow it—easily, pleasantly, and with results.

I don't want to overpower you with any clinical specifics, but as we go on and get to know each other better, I'll try, little by little to explain how my plan works, beyond the fact that it emphasizes a lower carbohydrate intake.

First of all, everyone needs carbohydrates in varying amounts. Sugars and starches are the source of our energy. Since they hit the bloodstream quicker than either fats or proteins, carbohydrates supply quick energy. The lack of carbohydrates can lead to an ailment called ketosis, a form of acidosis which makes you feel sickly, upset and queasy. Since one of the big reasons you diet is health, you shouldn't fool around with anything that would even harm you even slightly. So we make sure we get our necessary supply of carbohydrates and maybe a little more.

Medical authorities agree that the daily minimum requirements are sixty grams of carbohydrates. Figuring four calories to a gram we should aim at a minimum daily carbo-cal intake of 250 or so.

Proteins and fats are the other food essentials. They supply the fuel that sustains our blood sugar level which gives us staying power.

For any diet to be successful, the dieter has to want to lose weight badly enough to change his eating habits. And he has to use some common sense in the way he goes about removing surplus weight. If quite overweight, he should check with a doctor. He must be willing to undergo some sacrifice, but not to the degree that he will consider himself a martyr and reward himself with nineteen cookies for being good twenty consecutive minutes.

I make no boasts at all about my plan being one of those "fun" diets that will cause you to shed pounds miraculously overnight. You've seen those ads. My plan does require some discipline, some self-control. However, it's versatile, satisfying, and nutritious enough so that after you're into it for a while, it won't feel like a diet at all. Rather it will feel like a system of eating and drinking that's effective and lasting. You'll lose weight with it, which is the reason you're on it in the first place.

According to recent statistics, nearly seventy million Americans are overweight. They spend $100 million a year trying to lose weight. That's not counting how much they spent getting the poundage on to begin with. If you work it right, the dough you lay out for this volume will be all you will ever contribute to the weight reduction industry.

3.
The Potato Plot

I love flying. Always have. Even before I became a pilot with the Marines. Even while I *was* a pilot with the Marines. I have a job that takes me to places like Denmark, Acapulco, Florida, not to mention the unmentionable (and uncountable) flights to the West Coast with the "Tonight Show." All of which means that I probably log about 150,000 air miles a year. Still, I love flying. There's only one thing against flying. It's dangerous . . . because of all that good food they hand out.

Ever read those menus? If King Henry the Eighth were around he'd be flying all the time, just to sample the wines. And then there are those desserts that airlines love to serve, and all that other stuff that can really hi-jack the most determined weight-dropper off his diet. And of all the rich foods they lay on you, the most rapacious enemy to thinking thin is the common potato.

As I mentioned earlier, potatoes have been part of my life since childhood. Baked, boiled, mashed, home fried,

french fried, diced, parslied—everything. I'm a potato man.
Always been. Always will be. And it takes all my concentrated willpower to cut my spud-consumption by a
sliver. So there I am, travelling at six hundred miles per
hour thirty thousand feet up, and suddenly they lower a
pound and a half of those little flaky crinkled-up potatoes
into my lap. Can I, can you, say "No" to something so
heaven-sent? At least that's how it looks up in the sky.
When you've got your feet back on the ground—and your
head out of the clouds—you realize that air-borne root was
not the nice, juicy, steaming baked potato we all know and
love. What it was, was a rather tired, almost anemic-
looking potato that should have been sent to summer
camp to flesh out a bit. But that little wizened spud sitting there in my lap on the plane becomes my tormentor.
At home I could push it aside with a fork and forget it.
But sitting there in the plane, a little tense, more than a
little hungry (because I missed a meal racing to make the
flight), that potato baits me to the point of madness. I
feign sleep. But the potato knows. When I open my eyes,
there it is, right there, ready to become an excess part of
me. With each passing minute, the potato becomes more
and more attractive. So if you're a travelling man trying to
cut down your poundage, avoid being ambushed by the
potato. Reach for the cheeses instead. They're much lower
in carbo-cals and that's what we're after.

The dieter becomes food-conscious as soon as he boards
the plane and takes his seat. Pretty stewardesses are pushing appetizers and beverages and soon it becomes family
kitchen time.

You think food. You smell the aroma. You see others
eating. You try to concentrate on your next day's assig.
ment, but it's no good. Food wins.

It's time then for the pilot to talk over the public ad-
dress mike. Ah, there's something to divert you. Usually

he introduces himself and offers vital information about your altitude, speed and other factors regarding your flight. But with all the emphasis on food aboard, he might just as well be saying something like this to the man trying to reject the potatoes on his plate:

"Hi, I'm Smiling Slim Smith, your lanky pilot. I want to tell all you blubbery folks out there that on your plate right now is a potato that you've just got to love. Now this isn't your standard potato. Notice that cream in there and those funny flakes on the side. Doesn't look appetizing, but after all, looks aren't everything. Now that little potato there is good for oh . . . maybe 400 . . . 500 calories and countless carbo-cals. Take all you want. Eat up. Just sit back now and enjoy your flight to Suet City."

Flying east to west cross-country through the time zones you'll lose three hours, but you can gain three pounds. If you can't say no, I guarantee you that by the time you get to Phoenix you'll be flabby.

Potatoes and airmen somehow go together. Recently a group of American Air Force personnel attached to a wing in England were found to be woefully out of shape because they were over-indulging in that famous English standby, fish and chips. Fish is fine, but the potatoes were ruinous. It got so bad that the men were told to keep away from the British specialty and start taking off weight.

According to the USAF spokesmen, "If we were suddenly switched to a combat area, then overweight could affect our fighting efficiency."

And it could be pretty embarrassing for a portly pilot to be inserted into the cockpit with the help of three men and a large shoehorn.

I do owe a debt to commercial flying. It was on a plane that the realization came to me that I must go on a diet. I was flying back from a Super Bowl game and (between mouthfuls of potatoes) happened to look down at my shirt front. Don't ask me why. I don't know. Well, did you ever see those ads for Sanforized shirts with the big gap exposing your undershirt because you can't button the buttons? Right. I was the guy in the ads with the big gaps in my shirt front. I didn't care for that image. I realized suddenly that I was overweight. You get into a certain pattern of living and slowly but surely the weight imperceptibly piles up on your body.

It was then that I decided I'd have to change my way of living. I started searching for a diet that would help me get slimmer, stay healthy and active, and still enjoy my life. I experimented with quite a few eating plans and none of them worked until I came across this one. I feel it fits my life-style and hopefully, will be of aid to you, too.

At that time I weighed 243 pounds. At this writing I'm down to 209. By the time you read this I hope to be right on the 200 mark. And that's where I want to stay. So I manage to do pretty well in avoiding the starchy potatoes. I'll allow myself a lightly buttered medium-sized baked potato once in a while as a special treat. Believe me, when you desire something that badly and have it only on occasion, you appreciate it far more than if you've been having it right along.

Fellow passengers on plane trips do a lot to keep my mind off eating. People who recognize me stop to chat about a variety of subjects. If there is one general comment they make it's that I'm not really too fat and Johnny should "stop making those mean jokes" about me. The picture tube does exaggerate your size, adding anywhere from 12 to 15 pounds to your weight.

The stewardesses are lots of fun, too. When I sit down they'll come over and say jokingly that because of my well-known habits, the pilot said the two-drink limit on the flight doesn't apply to me. My public image has been firmly established by Johnny. When he says things like "Ed McMahon imbibes only soft drinks. Of course he considers anything you don't put into a car's radiator a soft drink," then you know you have a reputation to live down. So I stick to the two-drink limit and leave the flying to the pilot.

Racing for planes, schedule delays and stack-ups all can throw the dedicated dieter off his reducing regimen. Recently my manager, Bob Coe and I raced to catch a late night flight out of Kennedy Airport. There was a delay in taking off. We had gone without supper and were starving. We went to the restaurant. It was closed. We went into the bar, our stomachs growling hungrily in six-eight march tempo. They treated us royally, offering us all the drinks we wanted. Very nice, but we were hungry. I was about to start rapping my glass on the table prison-style and demand food, when one of the waitresses saved us from complete collapse. She went down to the employees' cafeteria and came back with two huge bowls of chili and lots of bread. Well, being as hungry as a pair of pack wolves, you know what we did to that chili and bread. I fell off my dieting wagon with a heavy thud, bruising my will-power and fracturing my self-control.

Eating at regular times to avoid getting ravenously hungry is part of any good reducing plan, although at times it is hard to maintain a regular eating schedule.

Another obstacle on the dieter's tracks while travelling is being recognized and given special treatment. Now that may not sound like a pitfall but it is. You're in Florida. It's late at night. There's no meal served on the plane you're to take. You're hungry, so you stop in at a restaurant near the airport. You finish a fine meal. You've done well. You trimmed the fat off your steak and enjoyed a substantial low-caloric salad. Now the owner recognizes you. He wants to extend a courtesy. So he sends over the dessert specialty of the place.

You know what dessert specialties are like. They're creamy, topped with nuts and cherries, gooey, syrupy and grow to a height of two-and-a-half feet. If it ever toppled over, a short waiter could get killed. Right there in front of you is about three months' worth of carbo-cals. It's placed there by your beaming host who insists you enjoy it "on the house." Now what do you do? You can't hurt his feelings. You have been going great diet-wise, but you have to at least sample it. Diplomacy will out.

So you try just a little bit. Just a taste. Occasionally you really get hurt because it *is* good and you *did* have a craving for something sweet and there goes your diet as you wade through the entire specialty. So, full and bloated, you climb aboard the plane for the flight back home. The airlines advertise more leg room. They should advertise more stomach room for the over-eater.

Everyone goes off diets from time to time. The idea is not to stay off, to get back on as soon as possible. Eating binges will slow your weight loss, but they aren't necessarily destructive if your diet is palatable and enjoyable.

Harvard nutritionist Dr. Frederick Stare says, "Overweight results not from what you eat and drink between Christmas and New Year's, but from what you eat and drink between New Year's and Christmas." That just about says it. That's why your eating plan must be a good, all-service, healthful, year-round regimen.

If you're constantly on and off dieting and your weight goes up and down that's not a healthy practice. It's called the "roller-coaster" and it can be harmful. When you lose weight, doctors tell you that your cholesterol goes down. But when you gain it back, for some reason it increases and becomes greater than it was before you started dieting. That's why a plan of dieting has to be one you can stay on with a minimum of dropping off for any extended period of time.

Diets based on fads just do not work effectively over the long haul, past records indicate. All diets arouse some controversy. They are either praised or deplored by the experts, the nutritionists whose business it is to know what takes off weight and keeps it off. They say that unbalanced diets—diets depriving the body of a vital amount of a needed nutrient—are unsafe and unworkable. I couldn't agree more. My cut-down carbo-cal plan is a *re*-balancing of your food intake. Americans in general eat too high a proportion of carbohydrates in relation to proteins and fats. Therefore, in essence, my plan is based on eating a smaller percentage of carbo-cals.

It has been thought, and generally accepted, that a calorie was a calorie whether it came from protein, fat or carbohydrate. But it is becoming more and more acceptable to believe that the carbohydrate calorie does the most damage. The first experiments on this were conducted in 1944 in New York. The tests, conducted by Dr. Blake Donaldson, included diets with a goodly share of proteins and fats with a lower intake of carbohydrates. The tests were declared successful and authorities began to consider the carbo-cal method of weight reduction. Further tests in England during the 1950's showed that people burned off more calories when they are proteins and fat calories than when they are carbohydrates.

Remember the basic rule is that if you burn off calories quicker than you take them in, you'll lose weight. If they burn off faster from proteins and fats, then it makes sense to cut back on the carbo-cals that take longer to burn away.

My program for rebalancing your eating patterns emphasizes the intake of proteins and encourages a reduction in carbo-cals. Another thing to consider is that proteins are the more filling foods. They'll stay with you longer and help fight off the stomach rumblings and forceful cravings for food that help weaken the strength of even the strongest-willed dieter.

Potatoes are rich in carbo-cals, therefore you have to watch them carefully. However they are inexpensive and plentiful and, most important, tasty. Breathes there a man with a soul so dead he doesn't go for French fries? But you must curtail the potatoes—not eliminate them entirely, that's too Spartan.

One cup (an average serving) of hash brown potatoes means 470 calories and 240 carbo-cals. Each French fried potato has 15 calories and 8 carbo-cals. A medium-sized baked potato is 102 calories, 80 carbo-cals. So potatoes can be rough. But there's no need to give them up completely. What you must do is budget your carbo-cal intake. If you have that baked potato, remember that you've taken in 80 carbo-cals. Your daily quota should be in the neighborhood of 250 carbo-cals, so you've got 170 to go. Keep that in mind as you eat your other meals or have that late night snack. If you have a potato or two during the day, it is advisable to leave the bread alone entirely and fill up on meats, fish or some low-carbo-cal vegetables. If you just can't resist bread, then go ahead, have a slice or two, but then leave the potatoes alone. It's a matter of give-and-take. You give up a little of the starch-filled high carbo-cals and you take off a few pounds. And you'll take them off consistently.

Vegetables are a vital part of our eating. No diet that eschews vegetables entirely is going to be too successful, or, for that matter, popular. The pivotal factor then is to find out which vegetables you should eat. Let's take a look at some of them and see how they stack up in the carbo-cal department. The best bets are spinach, mushrooms, cabbage, lettuce, string beans, turnips, onions and cauliflower, which was described not too endearingly by Mark Twain, who said that "Cauliflower is nothing but cabbage with a college education." Of course, Mark had no weight problem, so we'll put the cauliflower at the head of the vegetable class. There should be something on that list to please just about everybody. Any of these items can be eaten in good-sized quantities. You can even have second helpings without worrying that you are going to over-carbo-cal yourself. For instance, one cup of cooked spinach has only 46 calories and 24 carbo-cals. One compact head of lettuce has only 68 calories and just 18 carbo-cals. One cup of green beans contains 27 calories and 12 carbo-cals.

These are all first-line vegetables on the dieter's reducing express. There's a second group which contains slightly more carbo-cals, but not that many more to make you avoid them. Included here are kale, broccoli, Brussels sprouts and carrots. Now those two lists combined give you quite a selection to choose from. No need to get into a rut eating the same low-calorie food day after day as some specialized, concentrated diets insist.

You've got a wide range of healthful, tasty, nutritious vegetables to choose from to add to your dining pleasure as you go about the business of losing weight.

Also, there's enough variety to add color to your meal. Nutritionists and psychologists have long pointed out that the color of the meal, the eye-appeal has a lot to do with your enjoyment of it. Now I'm not suggesting you start tie-dyeing mushrooms for that mod look, but if you note the above list you'll see you can arrange a colorful combination of carbo-cal foods that will be attractive and delightful to the taste buds.

There are other vegetables in addition to the potato, that you should approach with a wary eye. These seemingly innocuous little items look innocent enough, but hidden in there somewhere are huge storehouses of carbo-cals just waiting to do you in. Be cautious about beets, applesauce (I include that as a vegetable because it is used so often with certain meats) lentils, dried beans, corn, peas and yams.

Again, there's no need to get rid of your favorite recipes that feature the above. Just be sure you keep your intake down to a minimum. Know that when you take a high carbo-cal vegetable you must atone for it by limiting your eating in another department.

It may be tough, but only for a while, because the choices are wide-ranging which precludes gustatory boredom, a wreaker of havoc among dieters. And, more important, there is so much variety available of fine food that it will become your new pattern of eating which will keep the pounds away permanently.

4.
Two Martinis
into Connecticut

You've probably heard about the commuter who stood in the train's bar car belting one martini after another and, as he finished each drink, he'd pick out the olive, place it into a small jar and order another drink.

"What are you doing that for?" asked a curious bystander.

"My wife told me to bring home a jar of olives after work and this is the best way I know. One more, bartender."

That's one way to shop, but a heck of a way to diet. I mean he wasn't putting those olives aside to save calories. For an olive, though considered to be dead weight in many reducing plans, is alive and well and sitting pretty as you please in the familiar pool of gin and vermouth at the bottom of dieters' martini glasses the nation over. Although each olive contains 10 calories, it takes two of the little fellows to constitute one carbo-cal.

So you see, when you hear a harried commuter tell you

that he lives "two martinis into Connecticut," don't think
he's fallen into bad weight-producing habits. For it's not
the martinis that do it, it's those vast collections of nuts
that somehow land next to your elbow when the wheels
begin to turn and you start rolling homeward.

I know a little bit about commuting. For seven years I
commuted daily to my job in New York from Philadelphia.
That's 90 miles each way. Think how many martinis long
that trip is. However, and I swear to you on a stack of
daiquiris, I seldom partook of the waters of life while
aboard the train. I used my time quite wisely. I'd hide
myself in a quiet coach, away from the bar car, and read.
It was one time in my life when I had the solitude to do
some heavy reading. During those years I managed to shut
my ears to talks about business deals and ladies in pink
hats discussing Broadway matinees to absorb such works
as *Barnaby Rudge, War and Peace, Anna Karenina, Bud-
denbrooks,* Hegel's *History of Philosophy* and Burton's
Anatomy of Melancholy. Actually I probably got a little
melancholy myself because I *wasn't* up in the bar car. But
I absorbed these works of literature instead of the potions
being served just a couple cars away. However there were
times when I put the book down to sip a couple to relax
and to observe the antics of the homeward-bound drinkers.
It was on one of these occasions that a near-sighted conductor missed my ticket and punched my *Moll Flanders*
instead.

Believe it or not, many commuters' wives applaud bar
cars; it lets the accumulated pressures from the work-a-day
world ooze out of a man's system so he can be hit afresh
with the accumulated pressures of his home.

A few drinks on the train at twilight keeps the working
man from taking the tensions of his job into his home.
There is a plan underfoot to install bar cars on morning

trains into the city so the man won't take the pressures of his home onto his job, but that may be only a rumor.

As in anything else, moderation is the key to the home-ward-bound drinker. Abstention can make the bar car work for you, as the wise wives point out, relaxing you, putting you in an amiable mood.

But I've seen some wild exceptions. On the trip back home to Philadelphia, there was one gentle soul who con-sumed a minimum of seven martinis. When he got off at the 30th Street station, he was floating nicely. His guilt always caught up with him then and fear set in. He couldn't face the little woman. To get up enough nerve for that ordeal, he'd stop at the neighborhood Happy Hour down the corner for a couple of drams of oral vaccine. Don't know what became of him, but I will say the last time I saw him he was quite slim. And one of the reasons, probably, was that he never dug into those carbo-cal cashews which were on the bar. By that time he probably couldn't even *see* them.

You may have hunger pangs on the train because it's been hours since your lunch. You settle back and have a drink. You relax a bit and those cashews and peanuts loom larger than life and twice as attractive. So you con-sider. Will you start in on them? The wheels roll out their rhythmic clackings. Somehow when you're hungry you hear those clackings as saying "good and plenty, good and plenty, good and plenty" and it helps to break down your resistance to the salt-drenched goodies.

Do your best to abstain, folks. Avoid this if humanly possible, for one ounce of cashews has 164 calories and 32 carbo-cals. And one ounce of cashews is hardly more than a cavity-filler at best. It's hard to stop copping cashews once you've begun.

Salt-stained nuts are put aboard bars to induce thirst so

the imbiber will buy yet another potion. Have the second drink if you will, but forego the nuts. That's the secret of not gaining weight on trains.

There's not much you can say about train food in general. The dining car on a train has never been known as a gourmand's idea of seventh heaven. Actually, I've eaten on trains a number of times in the past and it seemed somehow to taste like corrugated beaverboard festooned with strands of whisk broom. Not overly tasty, and not filling. So again, another trap is sprung—dessert. And there you go, slipping off your well-planned reducing program.

The railroads are getting better—*they* say. I read about the improvements and I'm happy, hoping only that the food improves along with the punctuality of arrivals and departures and the newer, brighter look in coaches and pullmans.

Eating meals on a train can be hazardous in itself. Not that you run into turbulence as you do on planes, but rounding hairpin curves at top speed while challenging a stew can be quite an epic struggle.

My favorite story along these lines concerns a neophyte train traveler who was ordering his first meal aboard the Super Chief. He sat down at one of those four-person tables next to a cranky old-timer who traveled regularly by rail. Our hero ordered a shrimp cocktail. On the first curve he let it get away from him and spill all over his seat partner. Upset to no end, the young man, feeling the amused stares of other diners, apologized profusely. The entree came, pork roast with gravy and assorted vegetables. Right. It happened again. All over the shirt, coat and pants of the veteran rail rider next to him.

This time the young man heard the amused laughter and was ready to throw himself under the wheels and end it all. People from all over the dining car were standing up to stare at him, thankful for this little divertissement which helped pass the time as the train rolled westward through the night. Our hero realized this. He had no intention of being center ring of this rolling circus. Still hungry—he hadn't eaten much of anything—he decided to dash off quickly and unobtrusively to the solitary safety of his little compartment. He stood up quickly and started off, as inconspicuously as possible.

But before he got to the door, the old-timer, still wiping away the pork roast debris shouted out shrilly to him, "What's the matter, fella? Ain't we having dessert today?"

Things like that can happen on trains, but commuters have their own special problems. The ride into the city is often just as harrowing an experience as coming home.

The trip cityward is often fraught with irritating delays, especially when you have a big appointment and you find there's a switch frozen somewhere in the Bronx and there's no way you can be on time. As sustenance against these nerve-blasting situations, you should never leave the house without a "good" breakfast. I put "good" in quotes because it is the all-purpose euphemism used to describe breakfasts. A man will say "I had a good breakfast today, but now I'm hungry again." Well, his idea of a "good" breakfast may be a lot different than a nutritionist's.

Perhaps the man had a "good" breakfast consisting of orange juice (four ounces), cereal with milk and sugar, and a cup of coffee. Well, that sounds "good," but let's step into the laboratory for a moment and analyze it.

A four-ounce glass of orange juice contains 50 carbo-cals. A wheat or bran cereal with milk and sugar contains 170 carbo-cals. That's 220 right there. I'm not counting the coffee, hoping that he takes it sugarless and black, not adding any more carbo-cals.

So that's one idea of a "good" breakfast.

Let's take a look at another breakfast. Tomato juice,

two eggs, four slices of bacon and coffee. The tomato juice (four ounces) has 20 carbo-cals. And guess how many carbo-cals for that hardy assortment of eggs and bacon? Do I hear 100? 150? No. There is only *one* carbo-cal on that plate. Letting the coffee go for a moment, your second breakfast contains only 21 carbo-cals, compared to the other breakfast of 220 carbo-cals.

Let's examine this a little more closely. Carbohydrates go into our bloodstream quickly, giving us a high blood-sugar level which we need for energy. But, according to tests by Dr. G.W. Thorn of Harvard, carbohydrates don't maintain this level very long.

After a high carbohydrate breakfast, "blood sugar rose rapidly but fell to an extremely low level, causing fatigue and inefficiency." And you know what happens when you feel fatigued—right. You reach for something sweet to satisfy your cravings. Something like a jelly doughnut during the mid-morning coffee break, adding another 120 carbo-cals to your daily quota.

The same tests showed that after a breakfast of skimmed milk, lean ground beef and cottage cheese, the blood sugar rose slowly to a high level and remained there for six hours. You are at peak efficiency without any fierce desire for something with satiety value in mid-morning. Say you eat that high protein breakfast at 7 A.M. and catch the train into the city to your job. You should be able to hold off easily until your lunchtime at noon or 1 P.M. without a crying need for something soft, sweet and filled with carbohydrates along about 10:30.

To me that makes sense. It's been effective for me and I'm sure you can see the logic in such an eating program.

The need for a filling breakfast should be obvious to all It is satisfying and comes at a time when you are about to launch into your work, providing needed fuel for your hardest efforts. The balanced diet, starting with a good breakfast, promotes good digestion, a vital aid to our overall effectiveness and well-being.

Writers, poets and philosophers have digressed on digestion.

From *Aesop's Fables* comes this note: "They found that even the belly, in its dull quiet way, was doing necessary work for the body."

More lyrical phrasing about the importance of a good digestive system is found in Joseph Conrad's *Under Western Eyes*. He wrote, "You can't ignore the importance of good digestion. The joy of life depends on a sound stomach, whereas a bad digestion inclines one to skepticism, incredulity, breeds black fancies and thoughts of death." Now that's telling it like it is.

Some people skip breakfast entirely, adding to their digestive problems and promoting an almost fanatical craving for some food in mid-morning. Still others have done the half-a-grapefruit bit on the theory that it possesses some magic power which will enable you to "melt away the fat" as some ads claim. But grapefruit is nearly 100 per cent carbohydrate, containing 70 carbo-cals out of 75 calories overall. And we now know just how long carbo-cals stay around to keep you moving at top strength and peak efficiency.

You've heard some people say "I don't eat breakfast because I'm just not hungry in the morning." Possibly it's true. But one of the reasons for this is that they overate the night before. And big meals before bedtime is the surest way to put on extra pounds.

In shaping your diet to help mold a new shape for yourself, it is advisable then, to start off with a solid breakfast—a "good" breakfast, one that is good for vitality, strength and reducing. Which brings up another point.

There are some people who don't know they are overweight. I was one of them. Fat sneaks up on you like a coyote in the night. Your way of living is set, but you just don't burn up the calories the way you used to before you reached the life-begins age of forty. In my case, I probably gained an almost miniscule pound every two months. Now that seems like practically nothing. But it adds up to six pounds a year. Spread that over five years (and over your body) and you're toting around an extra thirty pounds. Fat is insidious. It laughs its way into your heart and finds a home somewhere on your frame, usually in a most unattractive section like the waist or hips.

So how do you decide if you're fat. Well, I can tell you one thing—don't depend on friends. They're usually too nice to tell you. And you know the story about Bertha the Fat Lady, who weighs in at six hundred pounds telling Huge Hannah, "You're just right." Hannah weighs 390. Now that's heavy, but to Big Bertha, Hannah's just right.

The following chart lists the desired weight you should be for your height, depending upon your type of frame. The Metropolitan Life Insurance Company bets its bottom, profit-reading line on these figures so you can bet your next year's premium that these are right on the money. The desired weights are those that statistics have shown encourage greater longevity. The chart is for weight in indoor clothing for men and women twenty-five years of age and over. The height is measured with shoes on, one-inch heels for men, two-inches for women.

MEN

Height		Small	Medium	Large
Feet	Inches	Frame	Frame	Frame
5	2	112-120	118-129	126-141
5	3	115-123	121-133	129-144
5	4	118-126	124-136	132-148

| Height | | Small | Medium | Large |
Feet	Inches	Frame	Frame	Frame
5	5	121-129	127-139	135-152
5	6	124-133	130-143	138-156
5	7	128-137	134-147	142-161
5	8	132-141	138-152	147-166
5	9	136-145	142-156	151-170
5	10	140-150	146-160	155-174
5	11	144-154	150-165	159-179
6	0	148-158	154-170	164-184
6	1	152-162	158-175	168-189
6	2	156-167	162-180	173-194
6	3	160-171	167-185	179-199
6	4	164-175	172-190	182-204

WOMEN

| Height | | Small | Medium | Large |
Feet	Inches	Frame	Frame	Frame
4	10	92-98	96-107	104-119
4	11	94-101	98-110	106-122
5	0	96-104	101-113	109-125
5	1	99-107	104-116	112-128
5	2	102-110	107-119	115-131
5	3	105-113	110-122	118-134
5	4	108-116	113-126	121-138
5	5	111-119	116-130	125-142
5	6	114-123	120-135	129-146
5	7	118-127	124-139	133-150
5	8	122-131	128-143	137-154
5	9	126-135	132-147	141-158
5	10	130-140	136-151	145-163
5	11	134-144	140-155	149-168
6	0	138-148	144-159	153-173

Metropolitan suggests that girls between eighteen and twenty-five, subtract one pound for each year under twenty-five.

I know that when I read a chart like this I have a tendency to be surprised at how little the company thinks you ought to weigh. I'm 6 foot 3 and they suggest I weigh between 179-199. Well, I'm still ten pounds over the *highest* figure. My aim is to get below that. Ten pounds isn't too bad, but it's ten pounds too many. Well, it's better than nearly fifty which I was when I began my program.

Okay, let's say that you're pretty close to the weight regarded as suitable for your height. How do you tell if you're fat? If you feel some flesh jiggling unexpectedly when you jog or trot, you're fat. How fat depends on the kind of jiggling you feel. Let's say you're a non-jogger or that you really don't feel much flesh bouncing around. You should try the pinch test. It works like this.

You take your first finger and thumb and pinch alongside your chest, or below your shoulder blade, or on the back of your upper arm. If the skin you are pinching measures more than an inch wide, chances are you are overweight. The more skin you find yourself pinching, the more overweight you are. Five inches of fat being pinched represents a goodly amount of excess baggage you're hauling about.

At this time I might offer this cautionary word of advice. Try the pinch test on yourself. *Don't* try it on the pretty lady-friend of a burly acquaintance at a party somewhere. You don't add to your image if you come away mumbling, "I was just trying to find out if she's overweight."

Let's say that you have a good inch-and-a-half of fat between your thumb and forefinger. Let's face it, you have to lose weight. Even though you may be in the weight limits set by the charts for your body type and height, your frame is carrying excess avoirdupois. There are such things as overweight and underfat. Many professional athletes are overweight, but are not fat. Nutritionists are very careful to point out this distinction.

I'm assuming you're not a linebacker for the Minnesota Vikings, and so you figure you've got too much flesh on your body. You have to change your way of living. That's the big thing we're talking about. Not change it so that all the fun and games are torn away. Basically it's a change in thinking which will bring about the desired weight loss.

Another word of advice. Take your time. Don't expect weight to disappear as if Mandrake had suddenly waved his wand.

One overweight fellow went to his friendly neighborhood doctor and said he wanted to take off fifteen pounds. The man agreed with him and gave him a three-month program of eating and exercise.

"But, doc," the man protested, "I have to lose it fast. I've got a big date tonight." Wrong. You have to have patience and, as I stated earlier, a certain amount of willpower.

In any weight reduction plan there is what nutritionists call "weight plateaus." This is a level that the weight seems to want to stay at forever. Say you're on the low carbo-cal for a week. You lose three pounds. The second week you lose two more. You're going great. Now on the third week, you reach a plateau which is brought about by a readjustment of the water balance in your system. This third-week plateau is usually one of the severest pitfalls that the serious weight loser has to overcome. It brings about despair. What happened? I guess I'll never lose. And so you fall off the dieting and start eating too much again and the weight goes right back on.

So when you reach that plateau, don't give up. You know that it's there waiting for you. You simply grit your teeth and take it in stride, certain in the knowledge that if you continue eating as you had the first two weeks, the weight will start falling off again.

Now commuter or not, start your day off with a "good" breakfast, a meaningful opener as you start your day-to-day program to lose weight and add years and enjoyment to your life.

5.
Sitting Up
and
Taking Liquids

As I stated earlier, it's rough having a boss who keeps making snide remarks about my size. But I am caught on dilemma's twin horns. He is also downright uncharitable about my alleged drinking habits.

How would you like it if someone said things like this about you?

"Ed drinks quite a bit, but he never gets into trouble. Whenever he gets a bit noisy, the friendly bartender pours two warning shots over his head.

"Ed went for his annual physical today. The doctor found an olive in his bloodstream.

"Ed drinks martinis 8 to 1. After that he switches to bourbon and beer."

Now that isn't true. But it does, admittedly, make a handy launching pad for jokes. In fact, in my pre-show warm-up, a story along these lines gets me my biggest laugh.

I tell the audience that the stories Johnny tells about

my drinking are strictly rumors, "but last night that rumor came true. I went to my favorite place called The Library and I had a couple. I was, I admit, out pretty late. I started home about three in the morning and I was doing great. And then just as I rounded the corner, one block from my home, some wise guy came along and stepped on my fingers."

It is true that I will take a drink now and then, but it is not true that I am listed as an out-patient at Michael's Pub.

It is my opinion that drinking—as I use that word—is one of the joys of mankind's existence. Well-known figures of the past bear me out on that.

> *The man that isn't jolly after drinking*
> *Is just a drivelling idiot, to my thinking.*
>
> Euripedes, *Cyclops*

> *In the fruit of the vine, therein lies healing for all*
> *mankind.*
>
> *The Koran*

Drinking whiskey (from the Gaelic "Uisegebaugh"— Celtic for Water of Life) goes back to the early days of history.

I can just see the caveman who invented whiskey. He is mixing ingredients in a crude bowl and then tastes his product. He smiles. He leaps up and down. He yelps in glee. He's hit upon something. He offers a drink to his friend. His friend loves it.

"What do you call it?" he asks our primeval bartender.

"I don't know," is the reply.

"I don't know either," says the drinker, "but give me another and buy one for that girl down at the end of the cave."

It has been reported that the early Goths of Germany had the custom of debating everything of importance to the state, twice. The first time they debated it while all members of the council were drunk. The second time they went through it all again, this time sober. They debated drunk first so that the meetings wouldn't lack vigor, and then sober so that there wouldn't be any lack of discretion. Ever get the feeling our lawmakers do the same thing?

H.L. Mencken, the Baltimore iconoclast, once wrote that if every man had two drinks in the morning there would be no wars. If that's true I know quite a few people who are doing more than their share for world peace.

Drunkenness is abominable. But the proper use of alcohol is highly recommended to ease tension and soothe the rough edges of your nerve endings. It is said to dilate the arteries, which is the big reason many doctors recommend alcohol for older people as a weapon against arteriosclerosis. Statistics show that nearly three-fourths of the nation's adults drink occasionally. It is also reported that nearly one-quarter of adult men are heavy drinkers.

"Ed is a light drinker. As soon as it gets light, he starts drinking."

Now cut that out!

If you stop for that pick-me-up on the way home after work, take your time. Let the soothing waters do their job. If properly used, alcohol becomes a good friend. You feel a little better for it, a little surer that your life, after all, has some meaning.

Drinkers' stories abound and the one richest source is my all-time favorite performer—W.C. Fields. Here are some of Fields' most-quoted lines:

"I always keep a supply of stimulants on hand in case I see a snake—which I also keep handy.

"It was a woman who drove me to drink. And you know, I never even wrote to thank her.

"I always know when I've had enough—my knees start bending backward."

One of my favorites is the one where he walked into a

saloon for a morning straighten-me-out. He asked the bartender in that nasal whine of his:

"Barkeep, did I come in here last night, throw a twenty-dollar bill on the counter and proceed to drink until it was all spent?"

"Yes, you did."

"Whew, that's a relief. I thought I had lost it."

For all the stories of his predilection for alcohol, and most were true, Fields, according to his biographers, never really was so far gone that he didn't know what he was doing.

In other words, he stayed within his capacity, and to be wise drinkers we should all learn what our individual intake can be. Another thing about Fields, and this is where drinking is particularly important to the dieter, is that for the most part he drank a drink—lethal though it is—which contains only one carbo-cal. Right, the martini.

Now there are some drinks you can buy at your favorite place or make yourself at home which will lay as many carbo-cals on you as a rich dessert. A grasshopper, for instance, contains 235 calories, 72 carbo-cals. A four-ounce glass of port wine has 135 calories, 68 carbo-cals. A bourbon or rye highball with ginger ale reads 250 and 65, while a screwdriver measures 250 and 60. The biggest threat of all is the zombie, with 500 calories and 100 carbo-cals. These gamey concoctions head the list of alcoholic drinks you should avoid.

Alfred Hitchcock said he once weighed 365 pounds and went down to 200 by cutting out liquor and eating only steaks. I go with him on the steak part, but he really didn't have to cut out the liquor.

If you're not a martini man, try mixing your Scotch, bourbon and rye with plain water, on the rocks or with club soda. Water and club soda contain no carbo-cals. The calories contained in the drink are in the alcohol and they burn off quickly, sometimes as vapor from the lungs, according to Ronald M. Deutsch, writing in *The Family Guide To Better Food and Better Health*. This is especially true "when one consumes more than a little, as at a celebration."

He says from a "caloric point of view" it is better to consume a number of drinks at a party now and then, than to have one every day. He also added that his words *were not to be construed as a recommendation for periodic heavy drinking.*

Let's say your taste runs to vodka and gin with orange juice. Just switch it to a Bloody Mary, which is only 20-carbo-cals, a saving of 40.

Someone once asked me my three favorite drinks and why they were my favorites. Number one, of course, is a well-made martini. My second is a gem called Navy Grog. And third in my personal sipping sweepstakes is the little-known Galliom Stinger. Four of those and it's Wednesday all the time. Now believe me, those are strong drinks.

I think people often have too many strong drinks before dinner. I've seen people put away five martinis before going into the dining room for the meal. Well, sir, you do that and chances are you won't know if you're tasting beef kabob or a melted Hershey bar.

I recommend two good dry martinis before the meal. I say two because there really is no such thing as one martini. The only thing that will stop you before the second one is an earthquake or some other natural disaster. Actually, if you have more than two and you're not used to martinis, you may create your *own* disaster.

Two martinis will whet your appetite and sharpen your taste buds. And with the meal I've found it best to have what is termed an "adequate" wine. Be careful with the wine. Get to know them for their carbo-cal content. Generally speaking, the dry wines are much lower in this important department. Four ounces of Rhine wine contains eight carbo-cals while sweet Sauterne has 20. Four ounces of dry vermouth contains only 5 carbo-cals, while the same portions of sweet vermouth has 55, or eleven times as many.

I've mentioned why alcohol is good for you—it is a relaxant, it dilates your blood vessels and it helps to put you at ease in strange or unfamiliar situations. Now let me be fair and tell you how it can be bad for you.

Unless you indulge intelligently, you are threatening your liver. Alcohol can cause or exacerbate cirrhosis. It results in an increased amount of fibrous tissue entering the liver and impairing its function. The blood going to the heart from the stomach must go through the liver. No detours. These fibrous tissues serve almost as a dam to stop this blood and there's where you have trouble.

Now that's the worst it can do to you. And it can be very serious. The second worst is that when you are a known imbiber you are invited to cocktail parties, and these "parties" (so-called) are a no-man's-land in the battle of the bulge.

Some cocktail parties can be an exercise in fatuousness. They're often given by people trying to impress and you get 270 people in a room built for 130, all standing around saying the same thing. You know the kind. In the center of the room is a groaning board decorated with a novel centerpiece—like a potato salad figurine of Orson Welles. You eat and drink. Boredom sets in. You drink and eat some more. Oh, you can eat at these affairs. A cocktail party has been described as a place you go to tell how successful your diet is and gain three pounds while talking about it.

All cocktail parties, of course, are not like this. It's dangerous to generalize about anything, so I will say that I have attended some delightful ones and am available for more of the same. (Hostesses wishing to extend invitations, please contact my secretary and send photo.)

Some parties sparkle with robust wit and pertinent persiflage. One of the best lines I ever heard at one of these drink-'em-downs was uttered by George Gobel. It was one of those gatherings where a bartender strolled through the crowded room carrying a tray of drinks. Somehow the waiter had overlooked Lonesome George (George isn't one of our taller men) for an extended period of time. George, tinkling the icecubes in his empty glass, tried in vain to halt the drink-bearer. Finally he managed to throw a cross-body block to the swivel-hipping waiter. The waiter finally got the point.

"Care for another drink, sir?" the waiter asked.

"Does an accordion player wear a ring?" George replied.

Now I don't know if George had that one ready or not, but it really doesn't matter. It's a great line. Think it over. A great line. When cocktail parties inspire that kind of verbal lunacy then that's my type of party.

The biggest danger, of course, is the canapés. As you doubtless by now know, alcohol seeks refuge in our bloodstream and scoots right into it immediately after slipping by our tonsils. The presence of other substances slows down its hasty journey to its destination. Therefore, and this is advice handed down through the years, eat something when you drink. This, assuming the party-goer knows which alcoholic drinks contain fewest carbo-cals, is the pitfall for the dieter. At most parties you get the usual assortment of chips, peanuts, pretzels, finger sandwiches and sweet pastry bits. That's for openers. Avoid them at all costs. One dieter who couldn't find any cheeses or shrimp, managed to stem his impulses to reach for the peanuts by keeping both hands occupied. In one hand he held a Scotch and water, and in the other he had a tall slim blonde. He didn't gain an ounce and he made a new friend.

Assuming there's no blonde available, you'll have to use that free hand groping for food of some sort. Cheeses are your best bet. They are practically devoid of carbo-cals.

Check the cheese tables at the end of the book and you'll see what I mean.

If you can, divorce them from the crackers they may be resting on. Crackers are filled with carbo-cals. Or you might try shrimp or those tiny meat balls or frankfurters which have been run through with a colored toothpick. Stay with that game plan at parties and your good weight-losing intentions won't be shot down.

In addition to cocktail parties, the booze flows pretty free at a variety of functions—weddings, anniversaries, reunions. I don't really seek out celebrations, but I am a sentimental man and I end up at these affairs. There's always an anniversary sometime—somewhere.

For instance, my former secretary, Suzette McKiernan, worked for me a number of years. Every year on the exact date that I hired her, December 17, I take her out to dinner. It becomes an occasion in honor of a pleasant circumstance. When my present secretary, Pinky Coleman, returned to work after being ill, I gave her a little homecoming party to embellish the occasion. I do this and I can't help it. I enjoy it, and I don't really know why. Probably I have a deep desire to be liked by people. I've tried to analyze this trait and I think it may go back to my high school days. I was graduated with a class of five thousand. Nobody knew me. Nobody cared. I still remember those days as part of a particularly lonely chapter of my life. Maybe that's why I like to make events in people's lives significant and memorable.

And, of course, there are times when I have no one's homecoming or birthday or anniversary to celebrate. I look around and sure enough I'll usually find some occasion to celebrate. For instance, last week I gave myself a little party out of respect for the 20th anniversary of the deflating of the first Goodyear blimp. A good time was had by all. I served myself only cheese and tiny hot dogs and served myself only martinis, a drink I can honestly say I put together pretty well. Some have called it a real blockbuster. In fact, I won't serve you one of my martinis unless you have a note from your wife or legal guardian.

Everybody knows how to make a "perfect" martini, or else they're at least able to tell you why yours isn't perfect. There's an old story that says if you're ever lost alone in the desert, just mix a martini and some guy will be sure to show up and tell you how to mix it just a bit better.

Some formulas for creating the perfect martini might help. I offer these only to further the cause of dieters everywhere:

> •Spray a tiny bit of vermouth from an aerosol can over the rim of a glass filled with chilled gin.
> •Let the vermouth bottle stand by itself on the table. Then chill the gin and drink it straight. Your vermouth will last a long time using this method.

When I was in Korea we would pour the dry vermouth over the ice, pour it out again and then add the gin which mixes with the particles of vermouth clinging to the ice. My flying mates called it the McTini, but I cannot claim credit for its invention.

My favorite story is about the man who was home alone watching a pro football game on a Sunday afternoon. About 4:30 he got thirsty—and not a moment too soon, for it was martini time. He found two chilled glasses left from the night before. His pitcher was in the refrigerator, still filled with ice. He added the gin and vermouth and he felt a shiver of ecstasy course through him, a rapture that comes only once in a lifetime to creative artists. Here was the perfect martini. And not only one—he had enough of the mixing for two of them. Two perfect martinis!

Cautiously, steadily, hoping against hope that the taste would live up to its exquisite appearance, he took a sip from the first glass. Cold. Delicious. It *was* perfect. The greatest martini he had ever made. The greatest, in fact, that the world had ever known.

Then, as he stood there in the lengthening shadows of the quiet kitchen, a hand came down from heaven—and took his other martini.

That may not be true, but it should be.

But don't despair if your martinis don't evoke any celestial responses; just keep on trying. If you're a drinking man to any degree, it will help you in your fight to lose weight. Remember, it's only one carbo-cal a drink. If you're drinking them at parties, never lose sight of your goal—to take off weight. Keep your free hand away from the peanuts, potato chips and pretzels. And if the temptation gets too great, start looking around for that tall, slim blonde.

6.
At Last,
A Sure-Fire Way to
Lose That Weight

You say you want to reduce? You say you want to take off that excess poundage? You say you want to be slim and trim so perfect strangers on the street will stop you and say, "Hey, you're slim and trim?" Tell you what I'm gonna do. I'm gonna suggest you go out and get a scale.

Pitchman talk aside, the basic step on your path to weight reduction is to get a scale. You should weigh yourself daily. If that's impossible for any reason (I'm not one to pry) then certainly twice a week at least. The importance of this aspect of your battle to get slim and stay that way is borne out by a practice of the Sterling Drug Co. executives in New York. Each weekday at noon the firm's thinking men get weighed. They record the weight on a wall chart. A gain of two pounds calls for a warning. Three pounds and the man is banished from the dining room until he reverts to the desired weight. Rather harsh and militaristic, you say. Maybe, but it's proven effective. During the past five years only eight of the nearly eighty leading executives of the firm have gained as much as three pounds.

Dr. Irwin Stillman, who's been on the "Tonight Show" several times telling about his "drink plenty of water" diet, says you should weigh yourself religiously each morning at the same time. He states that a three-pound increase is as much a cause for alarm as a three-degree rise in your temperature.

Personally, when I'm home I weigh myself twice a day, once at night before retiring and once upon arising. When I first began doing this I thought I had chanced upon a new painless scheme of losing weight, because I weighed two pounds less in the morning than I did at night. Eureka, I screamed, (I do that occasionally) I've found it! A magic way to lose weight. You simply sleep your way to slimness. Alas and alack (I sometimes say that, too) it was only nature's way of letting your food find its proper spot on your body and become part of you, thus accounting for the loss as it assimilates. Anyway, the scale is an important asset if you're planning to lose weight.

If I had to pick a second most important item it's a mirror, preferably one of those full-length jobs. Friends sometimes are too polite to tell you. The mirror doesn't lie. If you're honest with yourself, no one need tell you that you're carrying that flabby inner tube about your middle needlessly.

A wall chart is a good idea, too. Another aid might be a tape measure. This is not only for our vanity. This will help you keep tabs on your inches-off program. Believe me, there's nothing as heady as knowing that your waist is three inches less than it had been, and that you have to have your clothing taken in. Great feeling.

Men, incidentally, have their toughest problems with the belly, just below the waist. Women find that fat clings to their hips, so that's their biggest area of worry. However, fat perversely hugs fast to all those extremities where it's likely to be least flattering, so regard it as an all-over enemy.

I'm assuming by now that you are acting on what I've been telling you and have started counting your carbo-cals and are aiming for about 250 of them daily. I'm not selling a thing except a way to get that weight off and keep it off. So pay attention, there may be questions later.

Now here's something for you to think about. A well-known New York doctor, Claude H. Miller, has kept score on how many people on clinically supervised weight-reducing programs have been able to attain the desired poundage and keep it that way for at least a year. Exactly *two* out of every hundred. You may be blasé about this, but that comes close to being a startling statistic.

So far I'm one of the lucky two. If I can do it, you can too. Your craving for the goodies filled with carbo-hydrates can't be any greater than mine. Why my plan is working is because it takes the pressure off my will-power. You can really dig into those proteins—eat a steak, or two if you can. Proteins are filling, they stay with you and often you find yourself so satisfied, that the enticing thought of a second steak isn't really that enticing after all. Again, I don't like my plan to be called a diet because it really isn't one. Also, I don't want you to confuse it with any of the myriad "can't fail, sure-fire" diets you keep hearing about.

You know the kind I mean. You may have tried one or two yourself. I have. There was the banana diet. For a while there I ate so many bananas I had nightmares of Tarzan carting me off to the jungle.

Fad diets are glutting the market today. Are fad diets valuable? Yes, says Dr. Philip White in *Today's Health* magazine—they're valuable for their promoters.

You've read about the way-out diets in many of the slick

magazines. Stop me if you've tried more than three of these: Continental Dessert Diet, Magic Formula-Plus Diet, Eat-All-You Want Diet, Revolutionary New Rockefeller Diet (that may include going to South America, getting stoned by unfriendly natives and losing eight pounds worrying about getting home safely), the Champagne Diet, Amazing Hypnotism Diet, Reduce and Stay Reduced the Egg Way, the Drinking Man's Diet, Apple Diet, Grape Diet, Mayo Clinic Diet (which, by the way, the clinic does not endorse), Dormitory Diet, Debutante Diet, Mother-Daughter Diet, Husband-Wife Diet, Wine Your Way to Slimness, the North Pole Slenderizing Plan (racing an Eskimo for a fish), Meat and Mushroom Diet, Eat Fat and Grow Slim, the Melon-Berry Diet, Hot Dog Diet, Snack Diet and the all-meat diet discovered by explorer Vilhjalmur Stefansson while exploring Alaska.

Recently the American Medical Association's Council on Foods and Nutrition called the Zen macrobiotic diet (particularly popular among the young), "one of the most dangerous dietary regimens."

The Zen diet a Japanese creation, consists of ten eating levels, starting with the "lowest," which includes a variety of foods such as cereals, vegetables and animal products up to the "highest," which is nothing but cereal. The theory is that when you subsist at the "highest" level you have then achieved a stage of "well-being."

The AMA's Council said strict adherence to the macrobiotic plan can result in "scurvy, anemia, insufficiency of protein and calcium in the blood, loss of kidney function, irreversible damage to health and [can] ultimately lead to death."

This is not my idea of "well-being."

There also are techniques of eating which have been presented as methods of reducing. There was a man called Dr. Horace Fletcher who introduced something called

Fletcherism. Dr. Fletcher had read that Gladstone, the British statesman, said every mouthful of food should be chewed thirty-two times. Fletcher was 220 pounds and stood only 5-foot-6. He started chewing his food far more than thirty-two times, turning everything into liquid, so nothing would enter his stomach as a solid. Reports have it that he averaged fifty-eight chews for a mouthful of mashed potatoes. Anyway, he lost 55 pounds and wrote a book about it. People took it up. In 1909 a leading magazine said that more than 200,000 American families practiced Fletcherism at the dining room table.

West Point instituted Fletcherism for its cadets. Army outfits tried it. A few colleges joined in. Finally the backlash came. Soldiers reported they were so weak from hunger they could hardly stand, let alone carry a gun, no matter how much they put into their mouths. Yale students, jaw-weary and tongue-tired from chewing, stopped eating meat and ate full meals of mashed potatoes and creamed spinach.

Then Fletcher began to cut down on his eating in a rather bizarre manner. He ate only potatoes, beans and corn bread. Then he decided not to eat breakfast. Then only one meal daily. Sometimes he'd go days without food. His teeth fell out and his resistance was so weakened that he finally died of a minor ailment — bronchitis.

I think I recall reading an article about a man who was quoted as saying "the chew-your-food-and-lose-weight" plan worked for him. He lost three pounds off his jaw. It may be just a canard.

I mentioned Dr. Stillman before. He's a funny, witty, intelligent man. I tried his "drink-all-the-water" diet. Not bad. Showed some results. But I did get tired of all that sloshing.

Dieting is a serious business. Clubs abound just for the purpose of aiding people who want to lose weight.

They meet to discuss their problems in sympathetic surroundings. TOPS is one of the best known. Take Off Pounds Sensibly is what the acronym stands for. They hold their meetings regularly and at each one, they line up and get weighed. The loss or gain is greeted by cheers and hisses. It works the same way, apparently, as Alcoholics Anonymous. In other words, you admit you have a problem, see that you aren't the only one with that problem, and this gives you strength to carry on. Chapters of the organization are all over the country bearing such names as the Zipper Rippers, Button Busters and Do or Dieters.

A while back I appeared on the Mike Douglas Show with Broadway star Karen Morrow, who told the nation she once lost 38 pounds through the help of Weight Watchers. One of the devices they used, she said, was to have a member come in from the butcher shop with a plastic bag of animal fat representing the excess flab the member took off that particular week. She found it a helpful gimmick. She took off all that weight and kept it off, as you can plainly see when she performs.

In addition to the various organizations designed to take off weight group-style, there are health clubs formed just to get people to go on dieting programs. One club in New York state reportedly has thirty-five different diets for their various patrons to choose from.

There are plenty of people who go there to reduce, and spend lots of money doing it. The diets may work. They may not. Again, possibly the only consolation is that you meet people with similar problems and your tales of inability to lose weight don't fall on deaf ears.

According to the Metropolitan Life Insurance Co., 12 per cent of men and women between the ages of twenty and twenty-nine are more than 20 per cent overweight. That means if you're supposed to weigh 150 pounds, you are at least 180. That's thirty extra pounds you're toting around. Actually, you're working as hard as a mailman with a thirty-pound sack, but without those great retirement benefits.

If you think 12 per cent (one of every eight) is high, listen to what happens when Mr. and Mrs. America get older. Women first. In the thirty to thirty-nine age group, 25 per cent of American women are more than 20 per cent overweight; from forty to forty-nine the figure is 40 per cent, and from ages fifty to fifty-nine, exactly 46 per cent are more than 20 per cent too heavy.

Men aren't quite so overweight. From thirty to thirty-nine the rate is 25 per cent, the same as the women; from forty to forty-nine the figure is 32 per cent, and 34 per cent between the ages of fifty and fifty-nine.

So there you have it. Nearly every other woman and more than every third man between the ages of fifty and fifty-nine are far, far too heavy. If you are in that age group, start doing something about it. If you're on your way, whether in your teens or in your forties, begin avoiding ever becoming part of those depressing statistics.

If you're in this with me, I know what you go through. You're constantly sweating out the battle of the bulge day and night, rising to heights of ecstacy as you lose three pounds and dropping to the depths of despair as it comes back with interest, often compounded quarterly.

For a brief glance at the different reasons for dieting of men and women, a recent survey showed that 66 per cent of all male dieters did so for reasons of health. Biggest reason for women going on diets—48 per cent—was vanity.

There's no doubt about it. Dieting is tough. We're fighting life-long habits that sometimes extend back to infancy.

An article in *Parents* magazine stated that an estimated 50 per cent of boys and 80 per cent of girls were overweight to some degree sometime during the years from ten to eighteen. The article carried further enlightening statistics. If one parent is fat, the chances are 40 per cent the child will be obese. With two fat parents, the chances of the child being obese doubles, 80 per cent. You know with two heavy parents, there's got to be plenty of food around the house for the children to attack.

As I mentioned in Chapter One, there was always plenty of food around my house, particularly potatoes. That definitely had an effect on my eating habits.

There was also a period in my life that undoubtedly affected my eating ways. I was at a boarding school outside Philadelphia. The food was, to put it bluntly, bad. Institutional food can be unappetizing to say the least, but this place I was at could wreck bologna. And I remember getting badly scrambled eggs (they weren't really scrambled, just a little mixed up) on a pie plate. You'd end up eating a slice of egg, just as you would eat a piece of pie.

Harshest in my memory is what they did to liver. Strange doings. I remember force-feeding myself manfully, hating to look at my main course, the nasty-looking item resembling an unborn fielder's glove. I remember cutting it into smaller and smaller bits, smaller than bite-size, right down to swallow-size so it could zip past my mouth without leaving a trace of taste. Because of that experience I can't touch liver to this day, even though it is recommended highly by physicians and contains only a moderate 24 carbo-cals for a three-and-a-half ounce serving.

Paul Lynde, one of television's and movies' top funny men, had a weight problem stemming from his family's eating habits during his formative years. He says that he was thirteen years old before he realized gravy wasn't the meal's main beverage.

As you get seriously into your weight-loss program,

you'll hear statements pro and con about taking vitamin pills. I take a few pills while dieting just on the off-chance that a day goes by in which you don't get your full daily quota of the proper nutrients.

The anti-pill school's credo is to spend your money on food, not pills. The argument here is that if you buy all the good, healthful foods, your body doesn't call for any supplements. I'm inclined to play it safe where my health is concerned and if I take an unnecessary vitamin pill now and then, well, who's keeping score? I was glad to read that Dr. Robert C. Atkins, well-known New York weight-control specialist and leading exponent of the low-carbo-hydrate reducing regimen with hundreds of permanently successful dieting cases on his record, agrees. He suggests you take vitamins E, C and a B complex. Best advice, as always: check with your doctor and get his opinion.

Americans as a whole eat too much. We average about 3,200 calories a day. Only three countries top us in caloric intake. They are Ireland, 3,375; Argentina, 3,360 and Denmark, 3,255. But you must remember that people, as a rule, in these countries are far more active physically than we are in America. And calories burn away a lot faster if you're involved in physical rather than sedentary pursuits.

Biggest offender in pushing up the calorie total has to be sweets. America is the Big Daddy of sweet-eaters. Cakes, candy, cookies and ice cream are far more available here than anywhere else. In addition, holidays and special occasions bring out the greatest displays of high carbo-hydrate sweets.

I've been an offender. As a child I'd munch chocolate bars all the way through Saturday afternoon adventure films and serials which always left the hero about to fall from a cliff or about to be eaten by a platoon of poison-ous scorpions. You could gauge the excitement of the after-noon's film by the candy we ate. If it were a real good film it would be a three-bar afternoon. Sometimes you'd get a four-bar picture and occasionally you'd get a real winner and you'd eat five bars. Today, looking at some of the popular movies, you feel like rushing out and *visiting* five bars. But I digress. The candy eating, impulsive or unconscious, of my formative years stays with me.

I don't often have a craving for candy, but if I'm around the house and there's a Whitman Sampler nearby, I'll find it. And I'll sample them. And chances are, unless forcibly restrained, I'll keep sampling. A candy, like other items of sweetness, often is taken as a reward or a tension-breaker. I know when I stay strictly on a diet or try to go below the minimum requirements of daily food intake so I'll lose more quickly (a foolish habit, by the way) for a period of a couple of weeks, I tend to get a little tense. Maybe even cranky. I think that's only natural. My son Jeff lets me know he reads me by saying, "Oh, oh, here's grouchy home again."

I'm telling you the truth. I do get into these moods. But I'm from the school that says you never take out your irritation on others. Look, no one asked me to diet, right? If it does make me up-tight for a moment, we have, as humans, the free will plus responsibility to make a double effort to be pleasant. So I try to dismiss the stresses and anxieties which are corrupting my normal, take-things-in-stride manner. So I think pleasant thoughts and try to be nice and manage to pull out of it without offending anyone.

If I occasionally need help I'll reach for a martini to get me over a rough spot. Or a piece of candy. Remember, I said emphasis on willpower is reduced, not eliminated. I'm not perfect. I slip away once in a while. I'm assuming none of you are perfect either, or you wouldn't be in the same fix I'm in—battling excess poundage. Slipping away from your plan for a candy or other sweet is only a temporary aid, as it adds to your problem the next day or next week.

There's one great story about a woman who was desperate for candy. It was Sunday night and all the candy stores in her neighborhood were closed. She paced the floor desperately, craving for a candy. She searched her closet. Nothing. Her cupboard was bare. Then feminine brilliance won out. She picked up the phone, dialed Western Union and sent a candygram to herself. It arrived shortly after. Beautiful.

I can't figure out offhand how many calories are in a box of chocolates, but I can tell you that a one-ounce piece of chocolate fudge contains 115 calories and 92 carbo-cals. That's more than one-third of your desired carbo-cal intake for the day. All your popular candy bars run between 60 and 100 carbo-cals, and just a plain marshmallow has 24 carbo-cals.

Ice cream is probably the all-time favorite in Sweet Tooth City. Ice cream in all its various guises can set you back. I can do fairly well avoiding ice cream and frozen custard, but I have a slight problem here. My manager Bob Coe is an ice cream alcoholic.

Rumor has it that in his office wall safe, he keeps a detailed map showing the exact locations of all the Baskin-Robbins ice cream parlors across the country. When we're travelling and have dinner out together, he never fails to top it off with some gooey creation, mostly ice cream with a mad alchemist's conglomeration of syrups, juices and what is commonly known as "messy stuff."

Now that's Bob's personal weakness. And it can be a big one. But he does pretty well on carbo-cals because he'll cut down elsewhere from time to time to leave room on his intake chart for one of those mile-high melanges of frozen delights.

To give you an idea of what's inside those ice creams, one fudge pop has 318 calories, 90 of them carbohydrates. A cherry ice cream soda has 306 and 115. A scoop of butterscotch ice cream has 294 and 70, while a royal banana split, fountain size is the blockbuster—1165 calories, 400 carbo-cals! (It must be the Fountain of Trevi they're talking about.)

The third category of sweets that people reach for almost out of habit is cookies. Now these aren't nearly as devastating to your diet in comparison with candy and ice cream, but you should be aware of them. A Fig Newton contains 87 calories, 44 carbo-cals; an Oreo cookie has 52 and 30, while even the tiny animal crackers (remember them!) have 8 calories each, including 6 carbo-cals.

Now you're aware of what sweets can do, but there are times when you have an overpowering urge to have something sweet. A chocolate, a piece of cake, a chocolate chip cookie, anything. You feel you can hold out no longer and have to give in and boost your carbo-cal count.

But before you do, here's a bit of advice I found interesting and effective. It's from Dr. Morton Glenn who wrote in the *Ladies' Home Journal*, that if you feel a strong desire to eat a sweet, substitute a sour pickle instead. He says it somehow works to curb your cravings for a sweet taste.

It's worked for me on occasion and I can say that a sour pickle can sometimes sweeten your disposition.

7.
Metrecal,
Carbo-Cal and
Oh, Cal Cutter

Well, you can see by now that this is not one of those learned tomes, delving deeply into the workings of our digestive tracts or tracing the routes of a couple of string beans as they pass down into our belly. There is no "Dr." in front of my name nor is there a string of letters after it.

Also, as I'm sure you've already ascertained, this is not one of those happy-go-lucky little dissertations saying that dieting is a barrel of laughs and you can lose weight tomorrow night without missing a chuckle. What I'm doing is trying to relate person-to-person my experiences in fighting the weight problem, my constant conflicts and ultimate discovery of a successful eating regimen. I will try to pass all this on to you and I sincerely hope they do help in the war against our common enemy—obesity.

As I said, I'm no doctor and am not qualified to handle personal eating problems such as you see presented through letters in other reducing books. You've seen those letters. I've read many of the lugubrious laments describing the travails of being overweight and the inability to lose appreciable poundage. They're usually signed by a ubiquitous person called simply "A."

They usually go something like this:

> Dear Dr. Flarn:
> I gain 10 pounds a year and can't get into my dresses anymore. In fact, I have a hard time getting into my living room. Fresh kids post *Pass* and *Don't Pass* stickers on the back of my dress when I walk down the sidewalk. My boy friend jokingly calls me Volkswagen because he says I have all my weight in the rear. And worst of all, I eat like a bird. My friend Emma Scurly eats anything at all and she still weighs the same—398. But she's taller than I am. Any advice?
>
> Your friend,
> (signed) A

Now I don't know "A," but I have read her letter and many others similar to it while wading through pages of writing about losing weight. And I am sympathetic to her plight. I identify with it and I think I might be of some help.

People love to eat. We've discussed that. When psychologists get together and discuss food, they inevitably point out that eating is an atavistic ritual harking back to the days when families ate together, huddling close against the cold, the darkness, the unseen enemy. People love to sit down at the table and dig in.

About fifteen years ago some marketing men realized that the country was in the midst of a boom in self-consciousness about weight. Why couldn't they come up with a substitute for eating? Something good, something tasty, something hearty. Something you could drink easily, enjoy and avoid the tempting weight-producers that await you at the table.

And so Metrecal was born. Now Metrecal is fine. For any of you who might not have heard of it, Metrecal is a liquid composed of various portions of milk powder, yeast, vitamins, minerals and other ingredients which gave it consistency and flavor. It comes in an eight-ounce can containing 225 calories. The idea was to drink four a day for a caloric total of 900, skipping meals entirely, without suffering any loss of your needed nutrients.

Metrecal caught on throughout the nation. People leaped onto the Metrecal bandwagon. I was one of them. The product was well-publicized by movie stars, TV comics and politicians. If you remember in John F. Kennedy's 1960 presidential campaign he stated that seventeen million Americans went to bed hungry every night. Republicans replied, "Of course, they're all on Metrecal."

Sales boomed. Competition flourished as other canned low-calorie meal substitutes hit the market. The AMA's Council on Foods and Nutrition warned users against reliance on a dietary pattern that would not be permanent. Other medical sources pointed out possible drawbacks in subsisting entirely on canned liquids. But sales stayed high. Suddenly something happened. People got tired of not eating. They wanted to come to the table and enjoy their food bought with their hard-earned money. Many defectors said simply they were bored with the same routine of sipping four cans a day and eating nothing.

In the *Saturday Review,* writer Harry Golden asked, "Could the Greeks really have revered a Jupiter who drank Metrecal instead of ambrosia?"

Gradually people, including myself, returned to the table. Let me make my position clear. I didn't go all-out for Metrecal. I used it as a diet aid, substituting for one meal during the day, enjoying two others fully. But I guess basically I am an eater. If I substituted Metrecal for breakfast I would be left with a certain sense of emptiness, a dissatisfaction that nagged me through the day. Today for breakfast I'll have a pair of eggs and two strips of bacon. Practically no carbo-cals, far more filling, longer-lasting and far more satisfying. Besides, with the bacon and eggs, I know I'm *eating* something. It probably soothes some primal anxieties that go way back to the dark days of man's beginning.

But dietary products are still big sellers. People *do* want to lose weight. Many fat-fighters go to weight-loss specialists. Some of these aren't the most reliable practitioners, trading on a person's insecurities. There's an old saying, "The only thing that makes you more nervous than a bald-headed barber is going to a dentist who has bad breath." Well, you can add another bad news type—a 300-pound weight-reduction expert. Some of these do get fat in body and in wallet by preying on susceptible people who find they've suddenly gotten heavier and older looking and want to recapture the vitality and youthfulness of days gone by.

People love to eat well. Some eat tremendous amounts without showing it. Jack George, a tall, husky ex-New York Knicks basketball player could eat a meal with two or three steaks and all the trimmings and wash it down with a case—that's right, a case—of twenty four bottles of Budweiser beer. I've seen him do it.

Jackie Gleason is another known for his gustatory achievements. His consumption of pizzas and booze is legendary. A few years back Jackie went on a diet and lost more than fifty pounds. He keeps suits in three sizes, heavy, medium and reasonably slim. He keeps them all because his weight does fluctuate considerably making trips up and down the scale.

The pages of history are studded with fat folks. Abbot Mendel, creator of the Mendelian theory of heredity, was a fat man. So were Emperor Charles V of the Roman Empire, Dean Swift, Honore Balzac and Boccaccio.

King Henry the VIII was a glutton of the first water. Controversial tell-all author Frank Harris must have been some kind of trencherman because he wrote that he bought himself a stomach pump and after gorging himself at dinner "I pump myself out."

There's a famous story about the string-bean vegetarian George Bernard Shaw who was accosted on the street by a roly-poly confrere who weighed in the neighborhood of 300.

"Hey, George," said the chubby one, "from the looks of you you'd think there'd been a famine."

To which the playwright swiftly retorted, "And from your looks, you're the one who caused it."

Another witty exchange along these lines occurred a number of years back on the "I've Got a Secret" television show. A lady contestant came on and whispered to host Garry Moore that her secret was that she had gone on a diet and had lost 300 pounds. The panel couldn't guess it.

The celebrity guest was next with his secret. It was Orson Welles, who had been out of the limelight for a number of years and had grown exceedingly large since his last appearances.

"What's Orson's secret?" asked Garry.

Without a moment's hesitation, Henry Morgan said, "You *gained* 300 pounds."

People from all walks of life overeat. They do so for many reasons. Insecurity. Tension. Boredom. Some psychiatrists have gone so far as to say overeating is an emotional substitute for sex. I don't know about that, but I do recall hearing about a man who eloped with his refrigerator. However, I must admit that does sound like something from one of Johnny's writers.

It's not easy to keep from over-indulging at the table, particularly in today's society which is replete with available goodies. I always get a kick out of looking through the pages of some women's magazines. On one side of the page is a picture story showing how to serve pie a la mode properly adding hundreds of carbo-cals to your schedule, while right across from it is an article on the great benefits of a diet that can't fail to take off weight.

Let's face it, friends, dinner *is* an important part of our social and familial make-up. It always has been.

As Lord Byron wrote in *Don Juan,* "All human history attests that happiness for man, the hungry sinner/Since Eve ate apples, much depends on dinner."

Lord Byron knew his way around a dinner table, as he had a tendency to get quite heavy. He even came up with his own diet consisting of cold boiled potatoes and wine. There's no record of how effective it was, but I'll take the wine and let him keep the spuds.

From the *Anecdotes of Samuel Johnson* we read, "A man seldom thinks with more earnestness of anything than he does of his dinner."

We're clear on that. Dinner is important to all of us. But the important thing is, as with everything of value, use it, don't abuse it. It's tough, but I'll offer a couple of bits of advice that have worked for me and may work for you.

For one thing—eat before meals. A salad, a whole tomato or a stalk of celery will satisfy your desire for food, appease your hunger pangs, thus making you eat less when you sit down to the main meal. Do this about a half-hour before dinner.

What I've learned to do lately is to fill a giant brandy snifter with water (that's right, water—check it if you like) and ice cubes and sip it slowly. Try it. If water isn't overly palatable to you, then a large glass of a low-cal diet drink will do the trick. My particular choices are Fresca and Tab. On the subject of beverages (non-alcoholic) carefully avoid the general run you see all around you. They are bubbling with carbohydrates as well as with carbonation, as you'll see when you come to the soft drink chart at the end of the book.

Coffee and tea are two more weapons against eating too much. I got to the point where coffee made me nervous, so I switched to Sanka or Decaf. I take it straight without sugar. Some people use saccharine instead of sugar to cut calories, but there are many doctors, though agreeing that saccharine is a legitimate substitute, who try to keep the dieter from relying on any sweet taste in foods.

Another thing, and on this point I found complete unanimity among the doctors and health specialists I've read: Eat slowly. The up-tempo eater often finishes his food too quickly to satisfy his body's needs and thus reaches for more. Slow down.

One more thing—don't miss a meal. This creates an incredible craving in your innards which will turn you into a kamikaze eater when you finally hit that table for the big repast. Balance, moderation, abstemiousness are some of the key words to remember.

Let's talk about moderation while we're at it. We all go on eating binges from time to time. I do. My worst period is Thanksgiving. Great holiday. It was something the Pilgrims began for us to show their thankfulness that they survived the journey across the Atlantic and managed to live in the wilds of America. I wasn't at Plymouth when it started, but I celebrate it as if I were one of the founding fathers, stalking through the brush with blunderbuss at the ready, eyes keen and alert for the original sacrificial turkey.

I've discussed my Thanksgiving gluttony syndrome behavior with several acquaintances, and I found that I'm not alone. It is quite prevalent as a matter of fact. What happens to me is that I finish dinner, fully satisfied, filled to capacity. Couldn't look a piece of turkey in the face. Then, suddenly, something happens. I want more turkey. I try to wait until the fever passes, but it doesn't. Here it is only three hours after dinner and I want more turkey. I pick a moment when my conscience isn't looking, sneak over to the refrigerator, and like a thief in the night take out the makings of a hot turkey sandwich and go at it all over again. It happens every year. No matter how hard I try to cure my compulsiveness, I fail. I am helpless to withstand the blandishments of a Thanksgiving Day turkey and all the trimmings. Those pistachio nuts are part of the trimming. You remember I warned you against eating nuts at parties. Well, if I have one pistachio nut I'll have dozens, hundreds. And more. Just as there's no such thing as one martini, there is also no such thing as one pistachio. I plead guilty. They're *loaded* with carbohydrates. Don't even bother to look it up on the chart. It's a capital offense. But I go on and on, more and more, and hate myself the morning after.

When you go on a binge like this you *do* feel it the next day. You feel the weight on you. It makes you lazy and sluggish. Christmas time with its rounds of parties and family visits possesses much the same problems for us all. But for me, Thanksgiving is the Waterloo of my weight-watching.

After the binge is over (if we could come up with a catchy melody I think we'd have a hit tune on our hands with that), you try to compensate by eating less of everything. I don't have that "when I diet everybody diets" attitude that husbands and wives complain about. There's no need for it anyway at my place. No one has my weight worries. Michael and Jeffrey are in great shape. And except for brief periods during their teen-age years, my older two, Claudia and Linda never had to worry about what they ate. So everyone eats what they want except for dear old dad who has to watch most every mouthful. Oh to be able to retrain our eating habits without effort.

I used to be strictly a meat-and-potatoes man until traveling opened my eyes to a wide variety of cuisines, expanding my gastronomical horizons. Why I've even gotten to like Japanese food. In a moment of recklessness I even tried squid. I don't like it but my tastes have become so wide-spread that I'm now willing to gamble on anything when we go out to restaurants. I've learned to enjoy Greek, Polynesian and some Mexican foods. But even with these exotic dishes I try to keep an eye on my carbo-cal intake and not overload myself as if I were celebrating Thanksgiving in a foreign land.

Actually eating binges are not uncommon. Actor Roger Moore, familiar to TV viewers as "The Saint," slim and trim, admits to doing the same thing. He says he eats everything in sight for a week or two, puts on five to seven pounds and then suddenly reverts to his usual ways until his weight returns to normal.

People who perform in public are always concerned about their weight because it directly relates to that all-important "image."

Buddy Hackett, one of the greatest funnymen, has always had this tendency to go on eating sprees. Much of his hilarious material revolves around the eating or craving for food. Shecky Greene is another wild comic who worries constantly about his weight and occasionally he and Hackett have gone on the famed Duke University rice diet program. Durham, North Carolina, can never be the same with Buddy and Shecky turned loose at the same time.

Actor James Coco is always on and off diets. He'll go for a while doing quite well, then have a lapse. And he's got the greatest excuses for not sticking to his diet. "Had a pain in my shoulder this morning and had to eat something," he'll say, a look of stupendous pain invading his expressive features. Or, "I spent the morning trying on vests. Very upsetting. Had to rush out for some spaghetti and meatballs. Had to." (Sorry for tattling, James, but they asked me to tell it like it is.)

Many people, performers or not, take diet pills to suppress their desire for food. These pills are tricky. Most are stimulants. They can boost your blood pressure and heart rate. And eventually, it is reported, you can build up a tolerance to them, thus rendering them ineffective. Many doctors feel that most people don't need diet pills. If you feel they might help you, again I urge you to check it out with your personal physician.

There are many roads to travel in your battle to avoid rotundity. There's one story about an overweight man who failed at everything and, in desperation, went to see a psychiatrist. He had to stop overeating.

"Did the psychiatrist help?" asked a friend.

"He sure did. Now I do all my eating on the couch."

You may never have to go to a psychiatrist to curb your food intake, but millions of others try a wide variety of methods. Special diets, dietetic foods, weight-loss "experts," diet pills, reducing salons. Anyone trying one of those methods will spend a lot of money. You should ask yourself if it will be worth it. Will the results, if any, be lasting? I guess in the final analysis you should ask yourself one question before starting on a new plan: "Would I like to spend the rest of my life eating this way?"

Think it over carefully.

All the above aids may help—for a time. But in the long run you have to change your eating habits and you have to do it yourself. It may be difficult, but it's well worth it.

There are some unexpected rewards. Singer Della Reese who occasionally is guest hostess on the "Tonight Show," had been away for several months. She didn't know I had gone on my new plan. She looked at me, did a double-take and said, "Well, hello, Slim."

I don't know the rate of exchange on words for dollars, but that remark was worth plenty to me.

8.
How Many Push-ups Equal a Slice of Pumpernickel?

I've always been a physically active person. As a growing boy I was pretty good athletically, playing all sports
pretty well. At Boston College I was an end on the team
the year after Chuckin' Charlie O'Rourke led the team
to a victory in the Orange Bowl. My son Michael is a fine
football player and I got a big charge out of his gridiron
exploits for Bronxville High School. I hope he'll continue
to play in college. What I'm trying to point out here is
that I'm athletically oriented like so many men out there.
When you're younger and active you burn up a lot of calories to help stay slim and vigorous. And, now comes the
hard part, when you stop being so active, you often have
a difficult time cutting your eating down to coincide
with your caloric burn-off.

Many men just sit back when they pass thirty and let
that hard muscle and sinew turn to unattractive flab.
Believe me, there is certainly a strong temptation to do
just that. Think of all the great excuses you can use. Too

tired after a day's work. You have to take the kids some-place. Too much work to do around the house. Great show on television. Have to visit the in-laws. About the only exercise some men get is taking the garbage out and reaching across the table to spear another baked potato.

I know what that's like. It's the easy way, and I took it . . . for a time. Then I realized its potential harm.

It's not inspiring to look down and find that somehow you've developed a good-sized belly. As St. Jerome said, "A fat paunch never breeds fine thoughts." It also makes you look older and less attractive.

My lowest weight as an adult was 175 after pre-flight training in 1943. I was hard, lean and my waistline was correspondingly slim. I don't know what I measured around the waist, but I know it'll never be that again. But I do make every effort to get the waist into as good a shape as I possibly can. Of course, at pre-flight we had a fierce schedule of exercises. Today it wouldn't be advisable for me to even approach that rigorous a routine. But exercise is important for every one of us. Exercise alone won't take your weight off, but if you follow a good strict pro-gram along with your new eating plan, it'll help you to get back into shape.

My own personal exercise routine now includes two weekly visits to a gym. For an hour-and-a-quarter I do all sorts of sit-ups, push-ups to help keep my muscles firm. I also do various exercises such as head stands for grace, which performers constantly are aware of on stage. It also helps maintain good muscle and skin tone.

You've probably all heard of isometrics, which basically is working one muscle against the other. There are all sorts of these little exercises you can perform while doing other duties. You can, for instance, while waiting for that phone to ring, press as hard as you can against your doorway, really forcing your arms to work as if you really wanted to widen the doorway. Do not try this if you happen to work in a condemned building.

And when the phone does ring, tighten your stomach muscles as hard as possible, forcing them back as far as you can and releasing them quickly. Do this for ten seconds each time the phone rings, likening your automatic response to the Pavlovian method of reacting each time the bell sounds.

I, along with many people I know, share a dislike for riding in elevators. Not exactly a phobia, you understand, but it is quite discomforting for me to take an elevator. I avoid them whenever possible, but with my type of job I'm always climbing into one for rides as high as sixty stories. While I'm locked in that box I do the stomach tensing bit until the doors open and let me escape. It helps my abdominal muscles and also, just as important, keeps my mind occupied during the ride. This type of quiet exercise is what some people term "dynamic tension," making the muscles firm by tensing them. Some of these were included in the physical training program called the Royal Canadian Air Force Exercise Plans for Physical Fitness. And, as Aunt Blabby on the "Tonight Show" might say, "You get me a Canadian officer and I'll give *him* a royal exercise."

There are dozens of little tricks you can use if you can't get free to join a gym or take part in a supervised exercise program. Try tightening your neck muscles, or pressing your palms together as hard as possible. They are all effective and will work well for you once you get in the habit of performing these whenever possible.

All exercise is good for your body. Exercise stimulates the development of blood vessel tissue, including the heart's muscle tissue, which helps stimulate the flow of blood, easing tension and helping your body prepare for any stresses that may occur. And, as Dr. Kaare Rodahl pointed out in *Be Fit For Life*, people with unconditioned bodies are more susceptible to consequences of stress, such as peptic ulcers, skin ailments and heart disease. Moderate daily exercise will burn up superfluous fat, tighten muscles and help wear away bulges you don't want or need.

When we exercise we burn up calories faster. If you get rid of 3,500 calories, that's one pound. Now it stands to reason that when you're lying on the sofa gazing up at the ceiling you're not burning off as many calories as you would be when you walk briskly. Statistically when you simply recline, doing nothing except possible wondering if you should begin exercising, you'll use up 100 calories if you lie down for seventy-eight minutes. (If you do recline seventy-eight minutes, chances are you'll be fired and get plenty of exercise walking around looking for a new job.) If you walk briskly for nineteen minutes, you've burned off the 100 calories it took seventy-eight minutes to dispose of lying down. That leaves you fifty-nine minutes to try to get rid of more calories.

Walking is the simplest and one of the best exercises of all. We have become a mechanized society. A car has become a vital appendage. But so are our feet and legs. We should use them more and give the car a rest. Besides, you'll be doing your bit in the fight against pollution.

You're not going to slim down magically by walking. Someone once figured out that if you walk two hours every day and don't eat any more than usual, you'll lose a pound a month. Okay, now that doesn't sound like much. But carry that out over a full year. That's twelve pounds. It's the difference between weighing 168 and 180. If you're average height, that twelve pounds is the difference between a trim waistline and one that has a slight bulge. Walking should be high on your list of weight-trimming exercises. It's easy enough and you can't beat the prices.

Trimness and physical fitness were emphasized way back in the days of the early Greeks. The men of Sparta's army lined up naked every morning. Those who were developing even the slightest bit of pot belly were forced to do special exercises until they regained the uniform slim, trim look.

As part of his physical fitness program, the philosopher Socrates danced every morning. Now I don't do that. I *have* been known to sing a little in the morning, but not dance. However, I try to make a routine of doing five or ten minutes of various exercises just as I do at the gym. A radio playing some music is a definite aid in doing solo exercises upon arising.

The business of staying physically fit and not over-weight actually became part of a political platform in Denmark a few years back. *The Boston Globe* reported that a Danish Reform Party had, as a plank in its platform, a proposed law that would require citizens to hand over one hour's pay every month for each two pounds they were overweight. You can imagine the whirlwind of exer-cising that would have caused.

Let's look at some of the basic physical activities and see how many calories they use up.

Walking for an hour can get rid of anywhere from 270 to 350 calories, depending upon the speed of your walk. The faster you walk, the more calories you burn off. If you run for an hour (not to be recommended unless you are in good shape or have a doctor's okay) that's 800 to 1,000 calories taken away; dancing for an hour, 200 to 400; golfing, 300 (no fair riding around in a cart); skiing, 600 to 700, and tennis 400 to 500.

That gives you some idea of what an aid physical activity can be in your tussle with the scales. No matter what you do, you use up calories. The speed you use them up at depends upon the activity. Your daily routine will get rid of calories for you. An hour of washing and dress-ing in the morning (if you're on the slow side it can take an hour) will use up 120 calories. An hour of domestic work around the house accounts for 200.

These are the basic examples given by doctors and nutritionists when they explain the rate at which your body burns off calories. But there are some unique day-to-day happenings, particularly in New York, which hasten the calorie-burning process. I've jotted down a few of these occurrences and made an estimate of how many extra calories *I think* are burned off.

For instance, dodging a taxi driver whose rounding a corner in midtown Manhattan will get rid of 35 extra calories. A walk down a darkened side street after dusk in Manhattan and you see two men following you out of the corner of your eye—50 calories. A scream for Help—55 calories. A race for a cab against an elderly lady in purple carrying an umbrella—75 calories. Dodging slashing blows from an umbrella wielded by an elderly lady in purple who doesn't like to lose—100 calories. Well, you get the idea.

By the way, we're using calories here because they are the accepted unit of measurement. Our main purpose, of course, is to limit the amount of *carbohydrate* calories we take in. As we go along, we're learning the amount of carbo-cals in each type of food, so that we'll be knowledgeable about keeping our carbo-cal intake down to a daily average of approximately 250.

Exercise usually is a matter of habit and discipline. If you're accustomed to it from childhood, it is easier to do even if you've been remiss and have given it up for a number of years. We talked earlier of overweight youngsters. Naturally we all have known teen-agers who eat too much, but another factor in excessive girth among our nation's youth is lack of exercise.

As Jean Mayer, professor of nutrition at Harvard, and one of the nation's top authorities in the field, points out in *Overweight,* there is an entire deeply ingrained area of wrong thinking about exercise: "Probably no single factor is more frequently responsible for the development of obesity in adolescents than lack of physical exercise."

He points out that there is too much emphasis on caloric input rather than output. He also states that there is a widespread underestimation of the calorie expenditure while exercising.

Parents often concern themselves with getting something nourishing into their growing child while neglecting to apply the same care and attention into their offspring's physical routines.

Anthropologist Ashley Montagu states it succinctly when he says that "In regions where food is abundant, many mothers in the Western world do not consider that their young children are prospering unless they approximate a globe. Such a globular view of the ability to survive probably harks back to the time when food was less abundant and the focus of attention was on keeping children adequately nourished."

Another way of looking at the beneficial aspects of exercising is to consider that if you run for three minutes, you've burned up the caloric equivalent of a chocolate chip cookie. Or if you've got a swimming pool available, swim for thirteen minutes. Go ahead. I'll wait. There. You've done the Australian crawl for thirteen minutes and burned off a whole doughnut. If you look at it that way, it may help to bring home the value of daily physical exercise.

More and more doctors are recommending exercise. One plan that has gained adherents recently is the new pulse test devised by Laurence E. Morehouse, professor of physical education and director of the Human Performance Laboratory at the University of California at Los Angeles. He recommends that you increase your physical activity for the purpose of maintaining physical vigor and trimness and to condition your heart to be able to withstand stress and strain. The plan, as reported in *Reader's Digest*, calls for you to pursue an activity which pushes your heart rate to 120 or higher and "maintain that activity and heartbeat for 10 minutes or longer." He suggests you get your doctor's approval and warns against being over-eager, stating, "There are no added benefits to be derived from exhaustive exercise."

His various plans for improving your all-around health ranges from light calisthenics and pitching horseshoes to climbing stairs, rowing, swimming, pick-and-shovel work right on up to the more strenuous pursuits like basketball, skiing and mountain climbing. The idea is to choose something within your physical capabilities that are healthful and enjoyable.

Jean Mayer also points out another dieting and exercising misconception—that "An increase in physical activity is always followed by an increase in appetite." Not true, he says. I agree. But from what I've seen, our natural customs or habits seem to lead us to *want* to eat something extra. Possibly we feel it's expected of us for some strange reason.

That's a trap. But let's inspect that situation for a minute and accept the fact that we might fall into that trap. You've put in a good half-hour of physical exercise. You're tired. You take a drink of water. It's two hours until dinner. Water doesn't do the job of satisfying you right now. You pace the floor, opening and shutting the refrigerator, checking the cabinets, looking for something that isn't fattening, something that wouldn't negate all your physical effort. You reach for an apple. Right? Well, let's think about that for a while, checking the carbo-cal chart. A large apple has 160 calories, with 100 carbo-cals. How about a banana? Not good. A large banana has

120 calories, 115 of them carbo-cals.

Now I'm not one to put down Mother Nature's products, but we've come this far avoiding carbo-cals, so why ruin it now. You're hungry. You want something. But put that apple back and try a salad. You've got time, you have energy, so go into the kitchen and whip up something tasty for yourself.

How about a tomato and lettuce salad? A good-sized portion is only twenty-five calories, 20 carbo-cals. Other fine low carbo-cal salads you might go for include crabmeat, egg, chicken, tuna fish. That's a wide variety of tasty items that won't do your eating program very much harm.

Don't despair about using salad dressing. You've heard that they're all very fattening and since a salad isn't that appetizing unless you have dressing, then why eat something dry and not too appealing?

Let's discuss that situation. First of all, there are low-calorie diet salad dressings which you can use all day long without any disastrous effect on your carbo-cal count. But suppose there's something missing in these, to your taste at any rate, and you want that full-bodied, solid, thick dressing. Just go ahead. True, they have calories, but their carbo-cal content is very small and remember, it's the carbo-cals we're counting.

Check the charts at the end of the book for the complete list of salads and salad dressings you can eat with impunity when you come in tired from exercising and feel that you just have to have something to eat. Then check the chart of fruits. You'll have no trouble seeing the obvious differences in carbo-cal content. Then, go ahead and make your choice if you feel the need when hunger strikes about an hour or two before meal time.

9.
Thinking
Thin Man's
Thoughts

You've seen those ads—"will melt away inches of fat in two days"—"take a total of six to ten inches off your waist and hips just like that"—"trims inches off your waist, hips and lower back, without dieting"—"a new weapon against ugly fat." You put these all together and say them quickly and you'll have the start of one of Johnny's movie pitchman spiels parodying the late-night TV hustling hucksters from Hollywood.

They are, of course, all quotes from genuine ads for gimmicks ranging from inflatable plastic shorts, magic belts, body suits, undershirts worn by Buster Crabbe on TV, to exercise devices and "instant slimmers" designed to give your waist "sex appeal."

This whole field has popped into real prominence only during the past few years, capitalizing on the dreams of millions of people to get slim the easy way. Business is booming—more than two million Sauna Belts and Hot Pants have been sold through the mail since 1969—and the products involved are often in embattled controversy with many medical men who doubt their effectiveness.

Dr. Joseph B. David, head of the Clinical and Medical Devices Division of the Food and Drug Administration, labels many devices "pure junk" and says there is "no valid scientific evidence at all that they work."

Some of the gimmicks claim to make inches disappear off selected spots without even losing weight.

To this Dr. Sedgwick Mead of the Kaiser Foundation Hospital in Vallejo, California, says, "It is impossible to reduce waistline measurements permanently without reducing body weight."

Despite authoritative statements like these, the public still continues to buy all sorts of things that they feel will help them in their fight to lose weight. All these items do, it appears, is take a few inches off your wallet.

The AMA's Dr. Philip White states that today "People are able and willing to seek the easy way out," which is a big reason why questionable businesses flourish and people aren't able to keep the weight off after many attempts at reducing.

These belts and shorts designed to help you reduce come equipped with a booklet giving a fifteen-minute daily exercise plan. An early item was a plastic inflatable belt worn around the waist. Exercising while wearing the belt was supposed to provide a locked-in sauna-like effect to melt fat off the areas enclosed by the belt.

The "hot pants" which became about the hottest product in the field, have "thermal packs" filled with water which, it is claimed, generates extra heat from the exercise, which in turn will take away flesh.

There have been statements from "satisfied customers," but there are many who believe that it's not the inflatable pants that may take off inches, but the rigorous exercise routines that go along with them.

A spokesman for the AMA said people should be discouraged from using these devices. "It's ridiculous to believe that sweating—the production of a water secretion by the sweat glands—can get rid of fat, which is chemically and physically different from water."

Another doctor points out that you can put anybody into a hot blanket or sheet and they'll lose, but "When they start drinking water again, they will be right back to where they were."

While the inflatable shorts and belts were number one on the hip parade, weighted belts were second and maybe they tried harder. The wearer would strap on one of these devices loaded with ten or fifteen pounds of lead. The theory was that you'd work harder lugging this around and would burn off more calories. According to the *Reader's Digest,* a physiologist figured that you'd have to wear a ten-pound belt eight hours a day for forty-five days to lose one pound.

Now I'm just like anyone else. I wasn't really looking for a sure-fire way to lose weight quickly, I was just looking for an aid, some assistance in trying to take off pounds. I didn't go the Hot Pants route, but I did try a weighted belt. When my back started to cave in—well, that ended that.

Devices like inflatable pants and weight belts take an estimated $250 million out of customers' pockets each year. Manufacturers do not have to show proof prior to sale that the product is safe and effective. As Dr. Davis said, "Anyone can put a gadget on the market and make all sorts of miraculous claims, and then it is up to the government to disprove them."

This can take as long as five or six years while the manufacturers can make millions, he pointed out.

Methods of organized club-type treatment ranging from massage to sauna baths do countless millions of dollars worth of business each year. At the present time, the biggest rage in California is "mummification." Movie and TV stars of all shapes and sizes allow themselves to be wrapped tightly, mummy-style in a hurry-up effort to sweat off inches. After being wrapped, the subject is zipped into a plastic suit and feels he's wearing a "cross between a plaster cast and a corset two sizes too small," as a lady described it to a *TV Guide* writer who was there to do a story on TV comedian Marty Ingels getting "mummified." The "skin shrinking" process was developed by a physical therapist working with World War II veterans twenty five years ago.

The company, Trim-a-Way, guarantees you'll lose two inches the first session, and five by the fifth. The five-inch overall loss, according to the firm, will last three to four weeks before it's time to go back to get all wrapped up again in the fight against fat.

TV Guide reported that many big names are mummification aficionados, including Phyllis Diller, Shelley Winters, Eva Gabor, Hope Lange, Tina Sinatra, Jill St. John, Glen Campbell, Andy Williams, Sid Caesar and Henny Youngman.

I can speak only as a spectator regarding mummification, never having tried it, but I have taken what they call an herbal wrap while at the La Costa Country Club in lower California. They use a rubber sheet there and I imagine it may be somewhat similar to mummification. I was there two days and took off 11 pounds. But again, though that was satisfying, it is not weight that is going to say bye-bye forever. However, it does revive the spirit to see what you're capable of doing and it encourages you to pursue your new eating program.

Reducing salons with sauna baths and massages to pound the weight away are doing a thriving business throughout the country. Millions of American housewives, frustrated and unable to stay on a weight-loss diet, turn to these like a drifting schooner heading for a protective cove during a sudden squall. One story I heard involved a very hippy matron who went to her masseuse and told her to "take a little off the bottom."

The ads for these salons can't be accused of modesty in their claims. "Lose 10 pounds in 7 days." Or, "Size 10 can be size 8 and size 12 can be size 10." It seems to me that if a woman is a size ten or twelve, she probably wouldn't be in the salon in the first place.

Whenever I think of weight-reduction claims I am reminded of Al Capp's famous campaign in Lil Abner for "Mockeroni," a new food. "Eat like a swine and stay slim as a snake," was the campaign pitch. "The more you eat, the thinner you get." It turned out that the product was so good people could not stop eating it. So they got thinner and thinner and they ended up just floating away.

Whether it be sauna belts, Hot Pants, weight belts, reducing salons or mummification, the pounds and inches you take off are only leaving temporarily. As the old story goes, losing weight can be like losing homing pigeons. You think they're gone, and then you turn around and find they're in your own backyard.

You can take off weight permanently—but there is only one real way to do it. It's more difficult than inflating a pair of Hot Pants, but it'll get you thinner and keep you that way. You simply must adopt a new eating plan that you can live with. And, live longer with, as you'll see from actuarial tables on mortality rates of the overweight.

Oh, I know it's tough to change a way of living. It's easy to be seduced by some new magic formula. Look, I tried the weight belt. And I've been wrapped up in a rubber sheet to sweat the suet off. Pleasant. Relaxing. But it won't do the job permanently.

And when you're trying to reform it's doubly tough be-

cause there seem to be so many cookbooks leaping out at
you, urging you to try something new, exotic, and often,
weight-producing. Have you looked at your library shelf
lately or at the racks at your bookstore?

This brief list is chosen at random. You probably know
plenty of others. Among the tummy tomes are *The Dinner
Party Cookbook, Craig Claiborne's Kitchen Primer, Graham
Kerr's Galloping Gourmet Cookbook, American Jewish
Cookbook, Natural Food Cookbook, Company Cookbook,
Can-Opener Cookbook, Frozen Food Cookbook, The I Hate
To Cook Cookbook, Molly Goldberg Cookbook, Mrs. Man-
ders' Cook Book* (Mrs. Manders?), *365 Ways To Cook Ham-
burger, Casserole Cook Book, Freeze and Please Home
Freezer Cook Book, Settlement Cookbook, 10-Minute Gour-
met Cookbook, The Rolling Kitchen* (sounds like cooking
during a California earthquake), *The Peasant Cookbook,
Cooking of the British Isles, Quick and Easy Electric
Skillet Cooking, Wilderness Cooking, Bland but Good,
Allergy Cookbook* (Gesundheit!) *Art of Hungarian Cooking,
Cordon Bleu Cookbook, Scandinavian Cooking for Ameri-
cans, Chinese Cooking with American Meals, A Taste of
India, Red-Flannel Hash and Shoo-Fly Pie, Mystic Seaport
Cooking* and so forth and so on.

You'll notice there are cookbooks for all types of gatherings *(Company Cookbook)* all countries (Chinese, Hungarian), the handicapped *(Allergy Cookbook, Diabetic Gourmet),* and all situations *(Wilderness Cooking, Aphrodisiac
Cuisine).* Quite specialized. And it's probably not over yet.

I'm betting it's only a matter of time before you find a
whole new list of cookbooks that are highly specialized.
You'll probably soon be able to buy the *Escaped Convict's
Cookbook* (Food on the Run), *Hasty Dishes for Hiccough
Victims, Souffles For Short People, The Bunsen Burner
Cookbook* and the *People Who Walk Funny Cookbook.*
And when they appear it will only add to the conflict be-

tween the desire to lose weight and the urge to try new dishes and, therefore, eat more.

The fact that many people do overeat and have to be told by someone to stop eating has been recognized by numerous scientific minds. One of the more ingenious devices was reported a while back in *Control Engineering* magazine. It is a "pre-set strain-gauge circuit, mounted neatly underneath the shirt, to register abdominal tautness and start a warning buzzer in the pocket." What you do is tuck this little handy-dandy device among the folds of abdominal flab just before mealtime. As the overeater takes in food, the device registers the increasing tautness and when it reaches a certain point, the buzzer goes off, letting the diner (and everyone within a radius of fifty yards) know that he's making a pig of himself.

There are other methods to keep your friends and loved ones from overeating—methods that don't require batteries. For one, you can heat the butter knife. Or, you can serve coffee in rough-bottom cups to make the stirrer think sugar has already been put in.

But whatever we do, everyone overeats at times. And no matter what sort of plastic pants or weighted belts we wear, or how often we try to sweat it off or have it pounded off by heavy-handed masseurs, the fact is when we overeat, we gain weight. However, there are numerous foods which will allow us to eat heartily without adding much to our poundage.

As stated, I've always been a meat and potatoes man. But since I've changed my eating ways a bit, I've discovered a lot about one food that we take for granted—fish. It's a dish that I remember eating only on meatless Fridays, but it is something that should be eaten more frequently than that by any healthy eater who doesn't want to gain weight.

As Dr. Morton Glenn pointed out in the *Ladies Home*

Journal, "There is about a half-ounce more protein in a pound of flatfish than in a pound of choice beef (rib) even without the bone."

Fish is also lower in fat than meat. Broiled lobster is 1.9 per cent fat compared with a porterhouse steak which is 20.4 per cent fat. A mackerel contains a higher percentage of fat than other fish, 18.5, but this is little compared to a hamburger which is 47.4 per cent fat.

Since fish are lower in fats, substituting a meal from the sea for one from the ranch occasionally would have a beneficial effect on your blood cholesterol.

Salt-water fish are a great source of iodine. Shellfish like lobster, crabs, shrimp, are very good sources of protein.

Okay, fish are important healthwise. But how do they rate in our all-important category—carbo-cals? Right up near the top.

A four-ounce portion of bass has 180 calories and just a trace of carbohydrate. Three ounces of crabmeat has 90 calories and only three carbo-cals. A three-ounce portion of canned mackerel (the fattiest of fish) contains 155 calories, but not one carbo-cal. And if your tastes run to caviar, and if your pocketbook can afford it, go right ahead, for two tablespoons of Beluga buckshot carries 70 calories but only four carbo-cals.

Fish can be prepared in a variety of ways and, fortunately, the two favorite sauces of fish fanciers are tartar and Hollandaise. They both have next to no carbo-cals.

So may I suggest you hang up your weight belt, deflate your Hot Pants and start thinking fish more often. Make the fish meal tonight or order it in a restaurant, rather than letting it be the one that got away.

10.
Everything You Wanted to Know About Snacks But Were Afraid to Ask

I'm a late night movie buff. After I watch the telecast of the Tonight Show I'm often wide awake, so I watch a movie out of the past. The ones I chance upon aren't your classics. I watch flicks like "Ma and Pa Kettle Go Berserk," or "Bulldog Drummond Breaks His Tooth on a Bad Eclair," or "Fu Manchu Forgets to Say 'May I.'" You know the type. Now no one has tossed an Oscar at any of these films, but they do serve their purpose. They keep you mildly amused, sometimes doing double duty as a soporific. They also make you hungry.

It is these late hours that can become the bane of a dieter's existence.

There are times when the movie doesn't lull you to slumberland. It leaves you tingling with excitement and/or worry. You wonder did she make the right decision running off with the wart healer? Why does she frown so? Did her final decree come through? Things like that.

Now you're alone in the house. It's 3 A.M. A witching hour to be sure and all of you who've prowled the house alone while everyone else is asleep know what I mean. You want to sleep. Strike that—you *have* to sleep. Now, how do you sleep? You just can't wish and make it come true. And when you can't sleep, and you're restless, you are a sitting duck for that refrigerator, which, if you're fortunate—or maybe not so fortunate weight-wise—might have a duck sitting there ready for the taking.

Perhaps some of you humor fans recall the short film on trying to sleep made by another one of my all-time favorites, Robert Benchley. The man is restless. It is a few hours before dawn. Everyone else is piling up the Z's, snoring in rapt contentment. And Benchley lies there awake, tossing, turning, wondering about the capricious whims of fate that keep him from dozing off. His analytical mind ponders what sleep is all about.

First, he states, "Sleep is induced by the blood leaving the brain. Or, as in the case of alcoholics, the brain leaving the blood."

He considers taking a hot pine bath. Then he weighs the alternative—*not* taking a hot pine bath.

Finally he decides that his stomach needs soothing and that can be resolved only by a glass of hot milk. He gets some milk, heats it up and drinks it down. And then . . . .

"Don't forget to put the milk back in the icebox," Benchley reminds us. "Hello, what's this? What do you suppose this is? Cold lobster? Yes, yes, it is cold lobster at that. Might give it a try.

"Not bad, not bad. Ah, got a little too much that time. Well, that's all for tonight. Up we go . . . up . . . hello, what's that? Coleslaw. Ha! Ha! See that? Coleslaw! Yes, sir.

"Well, now, let's see what else we've got here. Let's see. Well, I guess I'd better use a fork on this.

"Um, hm, funny these things never tasted like this at dinner. Here we go. What's over on this side? A little chicken . . . a little chicken. Get some of that dressing in there. Oh well, I might as well be comfortable about it."

Next we see Bob seated at the table, a whole chef's delight spread out before him as he chews his way (hopefully) to sleep concluding, "Now this will fix up that insomnia, all right. On the whole, when using the hot milk method, it's better to have the milk brought to you by someone else after you have gotten into bed."

Often though at that hour, there's no one awake to get you the hot milk, so you must resort to the Benchley method of raiding the icebox. (For you youngsters out there, an icebox is an ancient device we once used to keep food cold. It was the forerunner of the refrigerator. It was smaller, squatter, and somehow twice as alluring.) I'm one of Carlson's Raiders when it comes to midnight thievery. I've raided the icebox so often there were times when I had frost on my head.

Stray and previously unwanted chunks of food take on an almost forbidden appeal in the quiet hours after midnight. As Benchley muses, "Funny, these things never tasted like this at dinner." And it's so true. I will say, studying what Benchley ate, that he destroyed only foods that were low in carbo-cals. Chicken, lobster, coleslaw. If you're going to be a snack sneak, best to do it that way. I often don't. I have to plead guilty to lifting a whole platter of cold spaghetti and meat balls. *Cold.* That's a pre-dawn taste treat and delight that no one has ever done a TV commercial on.

Also, a cold boiled potato, sitting there in its adipogenous glory, becomes as tempting as the ruby in the idol's eye in the movie about India. And I succumb too often. Not as much as before, but I still fall victim to the temptation of snacks late at night.

My favorite has to be cold meat loaf.

If Fu Manchu were trying to get a secret out of me, he

could try bamboo shoots under the fingernails or the Chinese water torture and it wouldn't work. But if he were to place a cold meat loaf sandwich in front of me, just out of reach, I'd strain and fight for it and he'd have me ready to tell everything I knew.

A short time ago my manager and I landed in Florida late at night. We went to our motel. I had eaten several hours earlier and since I had just gone on my new weight-reducing plan, I was quite conscientious about adhering to a sensible diet.

The restaurant and bar were closed, but the man and woman running the place were most hospitable, as I've found most people to be when you re traveling. She asked Bob and myself if we wanted something to eat. We told her no thanks. So she went into the kitchen and brought out a blockbuster of a martini. Two of those and you feel like playing "When the Saints Go Marching In" on the harmonica . . . whether or not you had a harmonica. Now, half-way through the drink and feeling a mite better I was more amenable to her suggestion that we eat. However, I still had strength enough to say no. The hostess disappeared into the kitchen and came back with a meat loaf sandwich.

I started to tremble. Here in the black of night somewhere in Florida, this lady had discovered my weakness, my soft spot. I really hadn't been too hungry, but the drink and the sight of that meat loaf turned me into a ravenous wolfhound. I was polite enough to hold off long enough to thank her, then I made that sandwich disappear very quickly, establishing a new Florida record for devouring a meat loaf sandwich.

At home or away, I'm a snacker. I end up playing refrigerator roulette. Out of six items in the refrigerator, only one isn't loaded with carbo-cals.

I'd like to give you a little test right here about snacks

and carbo-cals. Well, I warned you there might be questions.

Now I'm doing this for two reasons. First is to help you
save a few carbo-cals should the refrigerator try to win you
over tonight in front of the TV set. Second is to see if
you've been staying with me.

I'm going to list six snacks and you pick out the one
that isn't loaded with carbo-cals. Better still, see if you can
place them in the proper order—low to high in carbo-cal
content.

Ready? Here they are—liverwurst on rye, two large apples, tuna fish salad with a whole tomato, a dish of tap-
ioca, a three-ounce package of frozen strawberries and a
cream cheese-and-jelly sandwich.

Okay, make your list. I'll put the correct answers at the
end of the chapter. And no peeking. If you get them in
perfect order, you qualify as a carbo-cal colonel. If you get
the carbohydrate badboy at the head of the list you're sen-
tenced to thirty days staring at a potato.

Actually, once you've learned the approximate carbo-cal
content, you won't really go counting them off one at a
time. For instance, I know what orange juice contains in
the way of carbo-cals, so I just switch over to tomato juice
and save myself a goodly number of carbo-cals. I have no
sugar, candy only occasionally, and once in a while a
wartime ration of bread and potatoes. And also, I used to
love to do the bread and gravy bit—but no more. You'll
be able to approximate your intake. Just remember to stay
in the general neighborhood of 250 carbo-cals.

To meticulously count each calorie is always a stark re-
minder that you are on a diet. Changing your eating
habits is bad enough, but to be reminded constantly that
you're on a diet is damaging to the psyche and self-control.

The effect of strict dieting was best summed up by writer Samuel Hoffenstein in rhyme.

My soul is dark with stormy riot,
Directly traceable to diet.

Aside from avoiding desserts and starchy foods such as bread and potatoes, there is no time when you are reminded with such force that you are embarking on a new eating regime as snack time. A good definition for snack time is anytime. You know hunger, habit and temptation know no hour. However, a refrigerator and a TV set nearby present a formidable duo.

Oh, I know what happens when that real urge to snack hits you. You've held off for a while. You pace, you mutter to yourself and when you really get desperate, thoughts of sugar plums dance in your head. I've been hungry enough at times to approach the stage where you see visions.

I've had daydreams of a bunch of obese carolers standing on a corner singing "We Shall Overeat."

Alone at night, watching a movie, I've been swept up in thoughts about eating and dieting. Where does all the fat go that people lose? According to one estimate, Americans lose 250 million pounds each year! Now that's a lot of fat. Does it turn into a pollutant and waft into the atmosphere. Did your car fail to start this morning because of an unhealthy mixture of fat and oil in your carburetor?

Sure, Americans lose 250 million pounds a year. But how much do they gain? So your mind, locked with another dilemma, starts to wander as you grip the sides of your chair and grit your teeth to avert thoughts about eating.

Suppose a man gets a deep tan on his vacation. Then he returns home and promptly gains thirty pounds. Will the new flesh be tan or white? Thoughts like that drive me to near-madness. That's what happens when I get that long-gone feeling—I long for food, but I know I'm a goner if I submit.

And I'm not alone.

Recently Ruth Garvey wrote a humorous article in *TV Guide* detailing her inability to keep from snacking while parked in front of the TV set.

"The spicy meatball commercial starts me on the prowl; when Duncan Hines or Betty Crocker shows me a slice of angel food or a plate of double Dutch chocolate fudge brownie beauties, I think of Cass Elliot or Totie Fields and wonder if maybe I could sing or be funny. Doesn't do a bit of good. Out to the kitchen, back with a cream puff."

The dangerous part here is not going to the refrigerator, but what you come back with. A cream puff contains a lot more carbo-cals than a stick of celery, a small slice of cold chicken or turkey or yes, even my old bugaboo—cold meat loaf, which has 320 calories and 44 carbo-cals in a good-sized slice.

A loaded refrigerator, considered a sign of affluence in some areas—at least a sign of economic security certainly, is a conspirator in an underground plot to make our teen-agers overweight and undernourished, according to Mrs. Leanne E. Cupp, national vice president of the Future Homemakers of America.

When teen-agers—students and baby-sitters—are bored, "All roads lead to the refrigerator and malnutrition," she said.

Mrs. Cupp added that teen-agers eat at least one-fourth of their daily food intake in snacks.

"There is gum and candy all morning, cookies and potato chips in the afternoon, a sandwich, cake and soda at home after school and soda and pretzels with homework or TV after dinner—all empty calories," she said.

Boy if that doesn't present a true picture of too many American homes. These teen-agers, snacking away at all those carbo-cal rich foods, are tomorrow's adults and they should be establishing proper eating habits right now.

But snackers come in all ages and sizes. If you're a closet cookie snatcher, whether you're sixteen or sixty, the carbo-cals are doing their darndest to put useless and needless weight on you.

Some dieting specialists suggest you try this to cut down snacking. On your way to the refrigerator, stop and ask yourself, "Am I really hungry? Do I have to eat right now?"

Sometimes you can get a "no" answer to both questions without much trouble. So just consider yourself fortunate as you head back to the tube. But there are times you're going to get a "yes" and then what do you do? By the way, when you ask yourself if you're really hungry and do you have to eat right now, I suggest you conduct that quiz silently. Your family or friends might not understand your little monologue if they overheard.

Okay, I've asked myself the question. My answer is "yes" I'm hungry and I want to eat. My conscience argues a little, but it is no contest, for I am very hungry. So I'll open the door, reach for a celery stick, or a slice of white meat—turkey or chicken—(no bread) or perhaps settle for a cup of beef or chicken boullion. Some people can't have meat unless it's between two slices of bread. They'll argue that the low-calorie statement on the label of the loaf means they can have all they want. What it usually means is that the slices are thinner. That's your bonus lesson for today from the Jolly Homemaker.

If I'm in a munching mood, what I'll do occasionally is get a bowl and fill it with ice cubes—right, plain ice cubes—and chomp away as I sit there. It's like nibbling very cold peanuts. Of course, if some sneak came along and dribbled a few ounces of smoky Scotch into the bowl and threw it all into a tall highball glass I wouldn't argue too strenuously. But the plain ice cube bit works, as you'll see if you try it.

I hope a few of these suggestions help you in avoiding the refrigerator between meals, or as it is known in dieting circles, the snack trap.

Well, it's test time. Let's have a look at how you've done. Just hand your papers to Miss Freebish and I'll mark them.

	Calories	Carbo-cals
Tuna fish salad with whole tomato	140	16
3-ounce package of frozen strawberries	90	80
Liverwurst on rye	430	100
Dish of tapioca	260	180
Two large apples	320	200
Cream cheese and jelly sandwich	442	200

I hope you made out okay. Study the above and other foods for their carbo-cal content. When it comes to snack time it will help when you ask yourself if you're really hungry and your inner voice shouts back at you, "You know I am, Charlie."

Just reach for the tuna fish, chicken and yes—a slice of cold meat loaf.

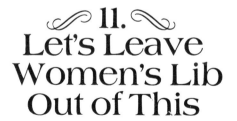

11.
Let's Leave
Women's Lib
Out of This

Hold it a second, ladies. Before I try to pass myself off here as a semi-authority on your particular weight problems, let me list some of my qualifications. First of all, I'm married. Second, I have four children and am familiar with all phases of home eating and the trickiness of feeding youngsters. Third, I can, and do, cook everything from simple stews to complicated repasts requiring hours of preparation. Fourth, well . . . I'm in favor of women—in general and in particular.

I know the daytime kitchen routine pretty well. The Old Man goes off to work and you're suddenly swamped by children rushing down the stairs asking for ties, the mate to a weird Argyle sock, spending money, bus fare. They also ask you to make their lunch. You try to avoid this. "You children are old enough to make your own lunch," you say, hands on hips. But you soon learn it's almost impossible for them to get ready on time *and* make their own lunch. So you do it for them.

Little Timothy sees you're making peanut butter and jelly. He complains. How about some of that leftover roast beef? No, sir, that's for supper. Well, Timothy doesn't exactly cry, but he pouts meaningfully, so you wink at your food budget and start building a couple of roast beefs. If Timothy gets one, then certainly little Denis and Donald should get one. This leaves you with a surplus of peanut butter and jelly sandwiches, one of which, at least, you will eat sometime during the day instead of that cheese or salad you had planned.

So the children are gone, leaving only their breakfast plates and the baby in his high chair, managing to get a good percentage of cereal into his mouth, but leaving an ample supply on the floor and/or the wall. So you clean off the breakfast dishes. There, that piece of egg looks good. And someone's cereal is only half eaten. Well, you can take care of that. Why throw it away? Now, you pick up the baby's dishes, scrape whatever tidbits might be there and you let him free. You then breathe a sigh of relief and sit down in the kitchen for your second coffee and possibly, just possibly, a piece of toast or sweet roll.

That scene is all too familiar. Your kids are going out into the world to face its manifold problems well-fed, which is the way it should be. But you sit home now, without having had a solid breakfast, but still piling up the carbo-cals from the remains.

In a little while it's time to do the food shopping for next week. You bundle little baby into the car and decide you don't have to make a list, but will be able to pick and choose as you cruise the aisles.

At this point I have to lodge a complaint. Why do women shoppers always spend five minutes jockeying their cars back and forth to get into the closest possible position near the supermarket doors? I've seen women grow old ungracefully backing up and pulling forward, adding wrinkles as they frown, straining forward to make sure their fenders aren't making intimate contact with a stranger's car.

A word of advice—park the car in the first parking space you see and *walk* across the parking lot to the store. You save time and you'll get a little exercise which we all can use.

I don't want to carp, ladies, or lose you as allies, but if I may, I'd like to suggest that you place your shopping carts in the enclosures built for that purpose. I speak from painful experiences. I had done the family shopping a while back and was loading about $48 worth of vittles into the car. As I bent over to deposit some chops into the back seat, a runaway cart, with rapidly increasing momentum as it raced down the inclined lot, wheels clicking madly, whammed me in the hip. Not the nicest feeling in the world, I remember thinking as I toppled head first into the back seat. I uttered a few dire imprecations at mankind (and womankind) in general and asked the patron saint of supermarket carts to spare me from further indignities. Oh well, they say you never see the one that gets you.

Okay, we've got you in the supermarket and you've made your second mistake, according to psychologists. You came in hungry. That's bad. It makes you susceptible to the blandishments of items you really didn't want to buy, but may purchase to ease your anxieties. Your first mistake? Not making a list. This makes you a target for the items that catch your eye and, importantly, may not be on sale.

Look, ladies I know it's difficult. When the piped-in music plays "Dancing in the Dark" with twenty-eight soaring violins leading the way, it's hard to resist buying the roast duck and all the accoutrements for a festive and/or romantic supper.

Then, ladies, most nutritionists agree that you should

spend more time reading the labels. For instance, say you're thinking of trying to take off some weight via the "dietetic" foods route. The word "dietetic" usually refers to low-sugar content. A recent study of chocolate cookies found that the dietetic brand contained nearly thirty more calories (and a commensurate number of more carbo-cals) per ounce than the regular brand.

Also, ice milk is not all that less in calories than some people might think. True, it is lower, but only about 30 calories per serving. So remember that if you think you can go wild on ice milk, believing you're not getting many calories and carbo-cals, that's simply not true.

You return home now, having bought several unnecessary items—that toothsome dessert for instance, and that bag of candy bars when baby began to wail near the checkout counter. After comes baby's midmorning milk and cookies. Naturally he doesn't finish. Just as naturally, you do.

Okay, it's lunchtime now and time for baby's nap. Oft-times housewives will get their babies in to sleep and then set up a little feast for themselves, possibly while finishing the morning paper or watching a TV show. These lunches range from bologna sandwiches to large hunks of fruit cake topped with ice cream.

As a man who's done this upon occasion, let me suggest a couple other noontime dishes you might want to try in an effort to keep your carbo-cal intake within the 250 mark for the day.

How about a tomato stuffed with chicken salad and a diet soda? Not bad. Practically no carbo-cals at all.

What about a tuna and egg salad platter along with a few chunks of celery?

Here's one you might like. A cup of chicken bouillon, shrimp scampi and a side order of creamed spinach, topped off with a cup of coffee. Now that's tasty, colorful, filling and it won't add much to your carbo-cal total. It will certainly tide you over until baby wakes up or the kids get home from school.

Ah, a word here now to you new brides. Now this is not a manual for newlyweds, but a few paragraphs of advice. Don't forget, fifteen years from the day you walked down the aisle, you're going to begin to wonder if you can still slip back into your wedding gown, just as the man will wonder if he is still slim enough to get back into his service uniform. Well, if you'd like to be able to do this, start now. Learn the good eating habits right away.

Many brides make one big mistake. Eager to show their new husbands how talented they are and how much they care for their mates, they overfeed him right from the start. Giant breakfasts, snacks, sweets, bread, rolls. We both know couples who've been married a year or two who've outgrown their clothes and have seemingly aged ten years in their brief married life.

These people, categorized as the Young Overweight Marrieds, are starting off life together cooking on the wrong burner. A woman thinks she's acting out of love, but it could turn out quite badly.

First of all, obesity doesn't make for romantic interludes. And, as famed nutritionist Adelle Davis says in *Let's Eat Right to Keep Fit*, many women bury their husbands early, just by overfeeding them. It's a simple method of doing away with someone, without the police coming in to ask embarrassing questions and dusting for fingerprints.

These are times when it is difficult not to overeat. Our society is such that, according to *Time* magazine, the average citizen can buy more calories than he can consume by spending only one-fifth of his income.

As Dr. Norman Jolliffe explains, the strains of overweight can damage the heart "for much the same reason that a Chevrolet engine in a Cadillac body would wear out sooner than if it were in a body for which it was built."

New brides should know this as they start their family meal habits, which can lead to obesity. You know the story about the man describing his wife of twenty-five years. "She still has that same girlish figure . . . only now it's hidden under twenty-five pounds of fat." Now we don't want that to happen, do we?

Where were we? Oh yes, the wife is in the kitchen planning the evening meal. A lot depends on her. Not only must she keep the family healthy, she must keep them *slim* and happy. She must close the edibility gap between her and the varied tastes of her consumers.

Let's face it. Some women cannot cook very well. I heard of one young housewife who is really bad. When she takes her turn at the stove she sends up so much smoke she gets answers from Indians.

Basically, when you cook, you start with meat. I've covered fish earlier and I hope you listened carefully. The meats are all-important, the most plentiful source of protein. Also, the most expensive item. The food industry, aware of this, has been working on synthetic products, known in the field as "meatless meat." At least ten firms are working on these, a type of product whose chief ingredient is the soybean. The bean is enriched with minerals and vitamins, and then colored and flavored to look and taste like ground beef, diced ham, chicken, sausages, etc. Although the government has already ruled that they can't be sold as meat and must be labeled with such names as "textured vegetable protein" and other equally unappetizing titles, the food industry has reported increased demand for these products.

Now they may be great. Probably are. But unless I'm forced to try it, I'll stick with the real things. To me a meal isn't complete (fish dinners excluded) unless some kind of meat is there. And although much beef is fat, meat basically is low in carbohydrates and therefore an asset in our 250 carbo-cal a day plan.

In the 1800's an English gentleman named William Banting, an undertaker by trade, tried for years to take weight off his 5-foot-2, two-hundred-and-plenty pound frame.

Banting tried everything. He visited doctor after doctor for help. No one could offer aid and comfort until he came across a Dr. William Harvey, who came, saw and concurred that Mr. Banting would indeed have to lose weight or he might soon be joining his customers.

Here is the diet Banting was given.

Breakfast: Four ounces of beef, kidneys, lamb, fish or bacon; one ounce of dry toast; tea without milk or sugar.

Lunch: Five ounces of fish or meat and any vegetable except potato; any kind of poultry or game; one ounce of dry toast; two or three glasses of claret, Madeira or Sherry wine.

Tea: Two or three ounces of fruit; a rusk or two; tea without milk or sugar.

Supper: Three or four ounces of meat or fish and a glass or two of wine.

This diet took Banting down to a far more reasonable 150 pounds. Banting, so impressed, published a book at his own expense and gave Dr. Harvey full credit. The world wasn't ready for this. How could a diet containing nearly 3,000 calories and so much fat help a man reduce? Harvey was denounced as a fraud. Banting was subject to much ridicule. However, Banting had the last laugh, living to the age of eighty-one and enjoying life a lot more since he took off that excess weight.

Let's take a look at this diet and you'll find one thing is quite obvious. It's loaded with meats, and fish that do have a substantial amount of calories, but are very low in carbo-cals.

The doctor recommended four ounces of beef. Well, three-and-a-half ounces of chuck beef contains 421 calories, but NO carbo-cals. Bacon, as we have seen, contains no carbo-cals. So you see this probably is the first recorded evidence that a low-carbohydrate diet, packed with proteins and containing some fats was effective.

Now if you'll join me in the kitchen ladies, we shall press on. First off, the method of cooking may have some bearing on the weights of those you're feeding. Naturally, frying and sautéeing are not as conducive to losing weight as boiling, baking and steaming. I'm sure you know all that as well, if not better than I do. Also on the market now are stick-proof pans which eliminate the necessity of using butter, oil or shortening.

What are my credentials for talking so authoritatively about your cooking? I'm glad you asked. I've been cooking since I was a kid. My mother and grandmother were excellent cooks. I enjoyed it from the start, because I was in control when I presided at the stove. Also, when you do that, you never go hungry.

Even today I'm an enthusiastic amateur cook. I just don't mean heating pizzas, I mean having the whole family get out of the kitchen while I prop up a cookbook and do the whole bit. If the recipe calls for something like dry mustard or endives that I don't have around the house, I get in the car and go out to get some. I go right by the book. It's an all-day affair, but dinner isn't until seven so I have plenty of time to make it come out right. One of my favorite cookbooks is movie star Vincent Price's collection of recipes. I can't wait until they make that book into a movie.

I love to cook meat. My favorites are roast loin of pork

with cinammon applesauce and carrots. A leg of lamb runs a close second, with turkey or capon third. Of course, I try about everything. And naturally enough, I polish off a goodly amount of what I prepare.

And there are times when I throw out the rules and ad-lib. I do OK in that department, too, if I do say so myself. And after parties, I'm always the gun in the kitchen making hamburgers or scrambled eggs and am pretty successful they tell me.

I have never gone to work preparing an armadillo yet, but I may tackle one next. Exotic food can be chancy, for as Swift, author of *Gullivers Travels,* said, "He was a bold man that first eat an oyster." He was indeed, but he must have enjoyed it. And that's the delight of trying new dishes. You never know when you're going to come up with some startling new taste treat your family will enjoy.

Always remember that the importance of hearty meat meals as far as we're concerned is that they are filled with protein for lasting energy and low in carbohydrates which put weight on faster and keep it on.

Another thing about carbohydrates you women out there should know is their effect on cavities. Many medical men state that carbohydrates have very little effect on children's teeth in the pre-eruptive stage, "However," says Helen Andrews Guthrie in her book *Introductory Nutrition,* "if the carbohydrates in diet replaces protective foods that carry nutrients such as calcium, vitamin D and vitamin C which are necessary for normal tooth formation, they indirectly have an adverse effect on the health of the tooth before eruption."

I think that's a point all parents should remember.

Women control things in the kitchen. That's where family weight planning begins. Sensible eating plans such as the low carbo-cal program can go a long way toward keeping your entire family out of the overweight class, or if some members are in that group already, do a lot to get him or her back down to normal.

At the back of the book, ladies, you'll find a group of recipes, all of which I've tried personally. I can guarantee their tastiness and beneficial advantages in our fight against excess weight.

Hope they help you to please your husband and family and in so doing make your marriage healthier and happier. Basically, I'm performing a wedding of low carbo-cal health and tasty nutrition—and that's my cooking story in a nuptial.

12.
Tension,
Anyone?

Any of you out there ever been in an earthquake? Raise your hands if you have. Stop trembling, sir. I was there, too. I was privileged (if that's the word) to be in California when the big baby of February 1971 struck. The "Tonight Show" had moved to the West Coast for one of its quarterly visits. We had been in our quarters at the Sheraton-Universal in North Hollywood for a couple of days when the earthquake hit.

I was up on the 17th floor when it happened, at just about six in the morning. Ever look out from a window that high and see the countryside shake and shudder and actually feel your hotel swaying? Not the most soothing feeling in the world. Your life flashes before you. You feel helpless and then, suddenly—lonely. Here you are ending your life alone in a hotel room 3,000 miles from home.

Well, they don't name earthquakes for girls as they do hurricanes, but if they did, this would be called Big Bertha.

It registered something like 6.5 on the Richter scale, and 8.7 on the McMahon Terror Scale.

I remember hustling into my clothes and racing to the elevator. Some of them had been put out of commission by the quake and the others were quite crowded. I don t like elevators to begin with, but under the circumstances I was happy to use one as a getaway car.

The doors opened and I stepped out into the packed lobby. Most of the hotel guests, including a good percentage of the show's staff were gathered around a TV set listening to further reports. There were several barefoot people who raced down without their shoes, while others had robes hastily tossed on over their night clothes. There was Doc Severinsen, his trumpet under his arm and three writers sitting together trying to put together some jokes for Johnny's monologue.

My first words in the lobby as I viewed the scene of muted panic were, "Cancel my order for that last drink, please." It got a big laugh and I guess that's about the best way to break the tension.

It was a quake that was a mighty force. As Johnny said during that night's monologue, "I want to announce that the meeting of the God Is Dead Club scheduled for tonight has been cancelled."

And, "It's an eerie feeling when you go to sleep alone and wake up in the same bed with a salesman from Duluth, one of Doc's saxophone players and a walrus from Marineland."

Now fear is the foster father of tension. After the original wave of fear leaves, you are left with a residue of tension. Believe me, the tension lasted the rest of the time we were out there because of the aftershocks. For days after the ground rippled, rolled and cavorted ominously under our feet at all times of the day and night.

It was an emotional hazard zone. When you feel the

first rumble you are supposed to look for an archway to stand under. Earthquake veterans say you do this because archways are the best-constructed parts of any building. For a while there I was tempted to walk around with my own personal archway, but then common sense prevailed and I took my chances along with everyone else.

Fear itself takes away your appetite, but it's not the nicest way to lose weight. Also, it's only temporary, because the ensuing tension and apprehension increases it. You are tense, your pulse rate is up. You are uncertain. If you're the type of guy who likes to be in charge of a situation as I am, the feeling of helplessness is tantamount to incipient panic. So, you eat and drink just a bit more.

True, that is a dramatic example of tension resulting from fear, but there are many undramatic day-to-day tensions that stimulate your appetite and make dieting that much more difficult.

Let's talk about these for a while. Today America, and the whole world as well, is in what students of societal life have called the Age of Anxiety. It is an anxious age, rough on the nerve endings and a threat to your peace of mind. This is true particularly for parents. Children today are exposed to outside evils that were unheard of when my generation was growing up. There is more affluence for one thing, and when people see more, they want more. The crime rate is frightening. The growing menace of drugs threatens the lives of many youngsters, who, at the same age a generation ago, might get their kicks by sneaking behind a barn for a quick puff on a cigarette.

The competitive nature of our society creates tension. The mechanization and computerization of tasks which formerly were manual in nature have created special emotional and psychological stresses that previous generations knew nothing about. The turmoil in world conditions is nothing new There have been few days in the history of society where peace prevailed in every land, but today our communications media have developed so much skill that they now can bring massacres from faraway places right into your dining room at mealtime. One doctor recently was quoted as saying that he considered watching a vivid news program a great source of stress. When these nameless fears gnaw at you, you seek relief, help, escape. Some people just give everything up and say, "Who needs it?" and hide someplace. Others drink. Still others eat excessively.

I go through the normal anxieties as often as the next person. Also, I have my own particular areas of tension which are peculiar to me because of the nature of my job.

For instance, I'm habitually punctual. If I have an appointment at 3 o'clock, I'm there five minutes early. I think somehow it's wrong to keep another human waiting for me. The person with a conscientious sense of time and/or consideration undoubtedly feels these pressures whereas someone who is casual in his dealings with people escapes that.

I live by the clock. I know that every day of the show the makeup man comes in at 4:30 P.M. to work me over. Each minute until I step in front of the audience a few minutes before taping time is rigidly accounted for.

After the show I'm often running for a plane. Let's say there's one out of LaGuardia at 7:30 P.M. I arrange my get-away with the producer, my secretary, my driver and manager and race pell-mell out to the airport. We arrive there just in time. What happens? Right. The plane is three hours late. Frustration. Tension. Anxieties. Sitting around waiting helplessly

As are most people, I'm a compendium of contradictions. For instance, I'm a pilot, have been one for many years. I don't like heights when I'm out in the open. I can fly an open cockpit plane upside down and I love it, but stand me up in an open area high above the ground and I panic. When we were in Italy a few years back, I climbed to the top of St. Peter's in Rome. I was there on a tour, a pilgrimage to see the famous sights, including, if I remember correctly, a view of Jerry Vale's birthplace. Anyhow, I went up to the roof but I began getting very nervous. Around the roof was a very unsafe looking railing. After all that climbing I turned around and went back in, pleading fright, insecurity, fear, you name it, and came right back down. I just couldn't do it.

There isn't a person around who isn't touched in some manner by the anxious tensions of our times. "Will the deal go through?" "Is my child all right?" "Will that lady in the red dress call me?" These are the questions whose delayed answers make people grow anxious and tense. Many people haven't learned to sit and wait and then accept the final outcome of any difficult situation. This leads to stress and frustration.

And there are other modern-day inconveniences and occurrences that create their own special brand of tension. I mentioned the McMahon Terror Scale. I also have a McMahon Emotional Stress Table, based on life's little ironies and fate's whimsical tricks.

For instance, if you're in a hurry and are driving behind a man who pokes along until he sees the light turn red and then speeds up, making the light while you get caught, that's stress. I rate that 8.5 on the scale of a possible 10.

I mentioned elevators. When you're plummeting down from the sixtieth floor and a sad-looking elevator operator begins singing "How Deep Is the Ocean?"—that's anxiety time.

If you're driving along the turnpike and a car passes you at 70 m.p.h. and a twelve-year-old kid points to your front tire and begins laughing, that's cause for worry.

I'm being facetious here of course, but only to make a point that life's daily happenings can provoke mental and emotional discomfort which can lead to overeating. A child can ask you nine times if he can go out and play in the blizzard and you take it in stride, refusing politely. The tenth time he asks may send you into a volcano-like roar that sends him looking for shelter. It happens.

Then there are all the things you feel you must worry about because you're supposed to. Ecology, pollution, endangered species, our forests, detergents, seat belts, David Frost's smile. Things like that.

The very real domestic problems which lead to frustration cause people to overeat. Dr. Ancel Keys, famed physiologist and health expert at the University of Minnesota, and inventor of the wartime K (for Keys) rations, relates:

> A fairly common experience for us is the wife who finds her husband staying out more and more. He may be interested in another woman or just like being with the boys. So she fishes around in the cupboard and hauls out a chocolate cake. It's a matter of boredom and the subconscious feeling that she is entitled to something because she's being deprived of something else.

People who write letters to doctors or editors of health and dieting books often complain they are always sick and troubled or in doubt about the state of their health. Very often, doctors point out, these illnesses or what the persons take to be illnesses are psychosomatic or emotogenic in origin. And there are, of course, the hypochondriacs who imagine themselves as having every illness ever known. I've found that many of them overeat to quell the tides of anxiety and morbid fears which confuse them.

They figure, "Might as well eat. What else can I do? Besides, when they take me to the hospital I'll get bad food." And they believe it at the time, although they can be perfectly well.

I remember a drinking friend who was always complaining about his health. But I never figured he was a true hypochondriac until one day when I saw him stirring his Tom Collins, using a medical thermometer as a swizzle stick. That's a worrier.

Smoking is what most people resort to when they want to relieve their stresses. I don't smoke. I think it is a very harmful practice. But many people do and that's another problem. Dieters who once smoked find that often they will gain weight because they snack incessantly the first few weeks until their system adjusts to the lack of nicotine, or until they satisfy their needs for oral satisfaction. The authorities are pretty well in agreement on that. However, since giving up smoking often leads to a few extra pounds, many people concerned about their weight often go back to smoking when they see their poundage increase.

Recently Ronald M. Deutsch in *The Family Guide to Better Food and Better Health* gave this answer to that problem:

> "The typical weight-gain of a withdrawing smoker totals about seven pounds, an amount not really difficult to lose. On the other hand, it has been calculated that the bad physical effects of smoking may be akin to those of carrying an extra one hundred pounds!"

So let's put smoking aside as a means to keep weight down and look into another method which I've always associated with soothing the nerves and lessening the stresses. And that is the old chicken soup method. For generations soup has been considered a cure-all for everything from scarlet fever to a sprained ankle. There's a great Jewish story about a man who'd been hit by a car. He's there on the ground, surrounded by spectators, police and the ambulance driver. A rabbi races up and says, "Quick, give him this chicken soup." The driver shakes his head. "Too late. He's gone. It can't help him." Says the rabbi, "It can't hurt."

There is a wide range of soups available to everyone who just may want to sit and sip and forget the cares of the day. But if you're working on the 250-carbo-cals a day plan, there are soups which can help and some which may hinder your reducing.

For instance, an eight-ounce cup of clear bouillon, chicken broth, consomme, has no carbo-cals or perhaps just a trace. The soups which are heaviest in carbo-cals are Navy bean (108), lentil (200), oyster stew (140), potato (100) creamed split pea (108). Needless to say, these are to be avoided.

Those are the extremes. But there is a big carbo-cal middle ground offering a lot of variety. These run from 20 to 90 carbo-cals. But remember, if you have a soup with over 50, compensate for it somewhere along the line by cutting back to keep your daily intake hovering around the 250 mark. Knowing that you've done that for a few straight days is in itself a help in calming ruffled nerves.

I'd like to inject a word here, particularly aimed at parents whose problems are heightened by the mores of our society—parents who worry chiefly about their children and the so-called "generation gap." As a father of four with an age range of pre-teen to mid-twenties, let me suggest that there always has been a generation gap and there always will be. True, external difficulties may be heightened, but the parent-child relationship remains the same.

Here's a quote I used when I spoke at my son Mike's graduation exercise at Bronxville (N.Y.) High School:

"Our youth now loves luxury. They have bad manners, contempt for authority, disrespect for older people. Children nowadays are tyrants. They no longer rise when their elders enter the room. They contradict their parents, chatter before company, gobble their food and tyrannize their teachers."

No, that wasn't a complaint made this morning by a harried parent. That was said by the Greek philosopher Socrates in the fourth century B.C.

So, you see, it's not a new problem. It's been going on for a long while. If that fact eases your day or lightens your load of tensions and keeps you from reaching for that extra piece of cake, then I'm pleased.

But meanwhile, go ahead, have that chicken soup. As the rabbi said, "It can't hurt."

13.
Your Health,
You Say

Ill-health of body or of mind, is defeat
Health alone is victory.

Sir Walter Scott

If it is well with your belly, your back and your feet,
Regal wealth can add nothing greater.

Horace

I like to start a chapter off like that because it makes one sound authoritative, knowledgeable. Actually, I *do* feel a little authoritative and knowledgeable because of the research I did compiling this book.

Another advantage of opening with a quote from a famous person is that it can give you a handy lead-in to a subject that is very vital, but one that can become grim.

That subject is health. Any time you start talking health, you have to consider the alternative—lack of health.

I remember several years back when an insurance sales-man called on me. He brought out a booklet showing a

147

happy, contented family seated around a glowing fireplace in a cozy living room.

He began his pitch, likening the pictured family to my growing one. Then suddenly, he slammed his hand down hard, covering the picture of the father and said, "Now just suppose you were suddenly taken out of the picture."

That shook me. But I can tell you that very shortly after, *he* was out of the picture. Let him scare someone else.

Actually, I can understand the salesman's dilemma. He's selling a product that gets to the very roots of our emotions—life and death.

I'm not selling life insurance, I'm pushing health. But in the course of that I must bring up a few statistics which are very relevant. I'm referring to the disproportionate incidence of mortality and illness in the overweight.

Bear with me as I press on.

"For each 10 per cent increase above normal weight, the mortality rate increases 20 per cent. Heart disease, kidney disease, strokes and diabetes occur two-and-a-half times as frequently among persons 25 per cent over normal weight than among those of the same age whose weight is normal."

That's from a book called *Eat, Drink, Be Merry and Live Longer,* written by Harry J. Johnson, M.D., who says overeating is "America's number one health hazard."

Gently but forcefully, the doctor goes on to say that sensible eating can become a habit ". . . and the resultant feeling of fitness can be much more rewarding than the temporary pleasures of lemon meringue." (A slice of lemon meringue pie by the way, contains 302 calories, 170 of them carbo-cals, about two-thirds of your daily quota.)

Science is constantly conducting studies on overeating. A short while ago at the Congress of Immunology in Washington, leading scientists suggested that mice "live longer and are less likely to get cancer if their lifetime food intake is reduced sharply."

Now I've never seen a fat mouse, but then I don't go looking for them. But I will go along with the men who feel that experiments conducted on mice bear a great relationship to, and contribute invaluable information about human life.

People do overeat. They go on food binges and then they sensibly catch themselves and go back on a weight-loss and maintenance regimen. The bad part is when the overeating becomes your mode of life. The insurance companies know what that can do to you and they let you know if you're willing to listen.

Here are a few quotes from the Metropolitan Life Insurance Company's statistical bulletin, "Overweight men experience a significantly higher mortality than men of average or less than average weight, and the greater the degree of overweight, the larger the excess mortality." Those words sprung from a thorough inspection called the "Build and Blood Pressure Study" conducted by the Society of Actuaries. Not exactly poetry, but you must admit it carries impact.

And we're going to give women equal time on this vital, if grim, topic.

From the same study: "In the age range fifteen to sixty-nine years, the mortality for women 10 per cent or more overweight was 18 per cent in excess of that for standard female risks; for women 20 per cent or more overweight, the excess was 25 per cent. The excess mortality rose steadily with increase in degree of overweight—from 9 per cent for women 10 per cent overweight, to 30 per cent for those 30 per cent overweight."

Okay, that's rough going. But sit back and ponder those figures for a while. And think about them again before you *do* consider having that lemon meringue pie.

Insurance people don't play fast and loose with figures. If you're heavy, you pay heavily to insure your life.

Recently Weight Watchers International, Inc., which has three million members taking its weight-reduction programs, has started its own insurance plan, applying the incentive approach. Members who take off the required weight and *keep it off* are given rate reductions. For example, a 5-foot-7 woman weighing 159 pounds (she's overweight) can get a $5,000 life policy from the American International Life Assurance Co. for $13.31. While a woman the same age (forty) who weighs in at 302 pounds (that's a lot of overweight) gets socked for $53.66 for the same policy. It's sort of a cash-for-calories recycling program.

We all know people who are much too fat. And they always have an excuse for overeating. I know a guy who has such a droopy belly he has to walk tippy-toe. He says he eats a lot because he hates his job. Well, it seems to me it's easier to switch jobs and change his eating habits. It could add twenty years to his life. If he doesn't some wise-guy cemetery representative will come along and try to sell him a plot in the elephants' burial ground.

Dr. Irwin Stillman, who, as I mentioned before, has appeared on the "Tonight Show" several times, is not a man to pull punches. He says succinctly, "I consider overweight the nation's No. 1 health problem. It impairs and kills more people than any other sickness. I believe it is vital to publish these proved facts because, shocking as it is, most overweights must *diet* or *die younger.*"

That says it. How straight-forward can you get?

Here are a couple more thoughts from Dr. Stillman.

"Lung capacity is reduced at least one-third because of crowding by fat. The liver is enlarged to one-and-a-half times its original size and is pushed up into the lung cage. The stomach is ballooned up to three times its normal size and pushes up into the chest."

William Shakespeare, who seemed to have something cogent to say about everything, wrote this about the fat man's excessive mortality rate: "Make less thy body hence and more thy grace. Leave gourmandizing. Know the grave doth gape for thee thrice wider than for other men."

We'll drop that now and go on to the illnesses the overweight are prone to suffer. High-blood pressure, hardening of the arteries, diabetes and arthritis are just a few of the ailments you become more susceptible to as you add pounds.

Recent medical reports indicate that the fat man has a 25 per cent higher death rate from cancer.

You see what you're doing when you stoke your furnace with too much food—you're hurting yourself and your loved ones.

Again, I must tell you that I am familiar with the joys of eating. And yes, even overeating. I've done that and I still do it occasionally. But I'm doing that less and less and it's paying off for me.

Our eating habits relate almost totally to our various life-styles. My particular way of life can best be described as weird. It's not your usual nine-to-five, thirty-five-hour week. I put in anywhere from fifty to eighty working hours a week. I'm on the go constantly. I get by on six hours sleep a night and occasionally sneak quick naps (That's *naps*, proofreader, not nips). I can doze off just about anywhere for a few minutes and feel refreshed. My one pitfall is Sunday afternoon. If I doze off watching a football game on TV, then I'm wide awake after that and finished sleeping for the night. In the main, though, those short cat naps are restful and contribute an awful lot to your general feeling of well-being.

I am (thank the Lord) in pretty good shape physically. I get periodic checkups and do as much walking and exercising as possible and stay in reasonably good shape considering I'm not out there sawing down trees to get more paper to write more books.

And, most important, I've managed to change my eating ways. I've learned to do without the things that pile up the carbo-cals on my hips, waist and other bad news neighborhoods. There's an old story about carbo-cals. They spend one second in your mouth, an hour in your stomach and a lifetime on your hips.

That's the thing we must keep uppermost in mind—cut down on those carbohydrates. Remember—250 carbo-cals a day.

Carbohydrates—starches and sugars—produce energy in our bodies with the unused portions left there as fat. When the proper amount of carbo-cals isn't made available, then the stored fat is used to give energy, reducing body fat and weight. It's as simple as that.

At least it's as simple as that in theory. It takes some effort to adjust and do something about cutting down the carbo-cals. But together, we can do it.

At this point I'd like to point out some of our most dangerous enemies. Anyone who wants to take off weight and keep it off must be aware of a pair of malefactors known as the two S's—standing for sneaky and sneakier. They are sugars and syrups.

Sugars, as I'm sure you are aware, are packed with carbo-cals. In fact, they are 100 per cent carbohydrate. Remember the days when you used to be able to go into the corner store and buy a square of maple sugar? Well, that was delightful, especially the way it used to melt and drip so enticingly. Fine occasionally when you're an active boy. But if you are an adult and sedentary, you should know that three-and-a-half ounces of maple sugar contains 360 carbo-cals. A simple little tablespoon of brown sugar has 50 carbo-cals. These appalling figures should be kept in mind by the woman who wants to bake a birthday cake. That's a lot of carbo-cals you're spreading around.

The same is true of the syrups you use in the kitchen. One-third of a cup of chocolate syrup has 250 carbo-cals, your whole day's quota. A third of a cup of corn syrup is even more devastating to your slim-down plan—300 carbo-cals. Again, keep these facts in mind when you're whipping up a festive delight for the family.

Avoid these twin terrorists and you'll find it easier to get slim, keep trim and stay healthy. We both want to be around a while longer. I'm sure there's no argument there.

14.
The Thinking Man's Diet

A while back there was a reducing plan which garnered quite a bit of publicity. You may recall it—the Drinking Man's Diet. Well, I'd like to give my plan the modest name of the Thinking Man's (or Woman's) Diet. Because, if you do stop to think about what I've been telling you, you'll agree that it can work for you. But admittedly, it does require some thinking.

Since we've come a long way together and I've laid bare all my innermost secrets (or almost all of them) about eating and personal life, I'd like to take it a step farther and tell all. (Look, if you can't tell your friends, who can you tell?)

I've mentioned some of my main weaknesses—meat loaf sandwiches, turkey, a good martini, etc., so you know that much about me. I've mentioned that a new balance of food intake, with emphasis on the reduction of carbohydrates would help you reduce while offering enough variety to take much of the pressure off your willpower and help you adjust to a new eating regimen as your way of life from here on. I also discussed the tensions of the day and the difficulties the type of job you have may present as you fight the good fight. Now I'd like to divulge my good side and bad, diet-wise; the black and white, good and evil, the Jekyll-Hyde dilemma that confounds and bedevils me. As you read on, I'm sure you will be able to identify with my conflicts and travails.

What I'm going to do is describe two weeks of my eating, including the high points and low marks. A good weight loss week and a bad one. Since I like to lead with my strong card, let's take the good week first. This was a relatively calm week for me. I went into the office about 10 A.M., and had no appointments during the week that kept me out after my stint was done with the "Tonight Show" at 7 P.M. Here we go.

Monday

Breakfast	—Half a grapefruit with artificial sugar. (88 carbo-cals)	
Lunch	—Glass of Tab (0 carbo-cals)	
Dinner	—Steak (trim off all fat) Asparagus Hollandaise (14 carbo-cals)	**Total 102**

Tuesday

Breakfast	—Scrambled eggs and two slices of bacon Sanka (4)	
Lunch	—Steak, hearts of Romaine salad with Roquefort dressing (5)	
Dinner	—Shrimp platter with Thousand Island dressing (4)	**Total 13**

Wednesday

Breakfast—2 scrambled eggs with Parmesan cheese
Sanka
(5)

Lunch   —2 Hard-boiled eggs (1)

Dinner   —Shrimp cocktail with Thousand Island
dressing. Steak
(40)   **Total 46**

Thursday

Breakfast—Half a grapefruit. Sanka.
(88)

Lunch   —Cheddar cheese omelette with bits of ham
(5)

Dinner   —Hamburger patty, green beans and salad
with Roquefort dressing
(32)   **Total 125**

Friday

Breakfast—Sanka (0)

Lunch   —Steak and Tab. (0)

Dinner   —Shrimp platter (4)   **Total 4**

Now that's really sticking to an eating plan. Look at
that. Only two of the five days saw my carbo-cal intake
top the one hundred mark. Admittedly that's a little low,
but I had had a fairly high week just before and I wanted
to make up a little. And I did. I lost a pound a day—five
pounds. Now a five-pound loss in five days is beautiful. I
felt very proud of myself. But before you paste any stars
on my crown, let me point out that all conditions in my

life and job were perfect. If my life were consistently calm and comparatively normal and free of occasions of cele· bration, I'd have no trouble maintaining that program. And once you do that for a couple of weeks, think of what a fantastic treat a cold chicken snack at midnight is. And you could afford it with ease.

Now that was the good week.

But now, enter the villain. Dark clouds gather, a strain of melodramatic music comes from the orchestra pit. I am traveling. I am away from home, catching planes, doing a TV special, spending all sorts of hours working and talking and planning. My day goes on for hours. Yes, friends, I fell off the wagon, succumbed to the pleasures of the road, the wining and dining, conviviality and pressures of dead-lines.

If you're going to take this trip with me, I must warn you to fasten your seat belts. There may be turbulence ahead.

My dark week begins, fellow food fans, on a Thursday morning. My plans for the next few days were all laid out neatly and precisely in the mind of my manager Bob Coe. I didn't know the exact schedule, but I knew I would be in for a hectic few days. As sustenance against what lay before me, I began the day with the perennial hearty breakfast, including an English muffin. The muffin alone cost me 120 carbo-cals, but I felt I needed it at the time.

At lunch I can't resist the breadsticks and butter (well, after all, I *am* traveling tonight and who knows what I'll get to eat later) followed by a small steak. In the late afternoon before the "Tonight Show" taping I have a bowl of soup and a cheeseburger. When the taping is done, I rush to the airport, have a couple of martinis on the plane, and a couple of those odd little sandwiches they hand out. There's a mimeographed Hogie in the middle of the menu, and I love Hogies. In deference to my diet, I take the top piece of the roll off. Before I quit I've eaten the entire Hogie plus the package of almonds that someone placed mysteriously alongside my martini.

We have a one-hour stopover in Atlanta and the hospitality of the airline lounge includes several handfuls of those delicious dry roasted peanuts.

We finally arrive at our motel in Cypress Gardens at 1 A.M. The owner and his wife graciously waited up for us and they offer me the Big Brother of that dreaded meat loaf sandwich I mentioned back in Chapter 10.

It's hard to believe I'm still eating on Thursday's time. I've consumed, let's see how many carbo-cals. The sandwiches, the Hogie, the almonds, muffin, breadsticks . . . well, my bookkeeper isn't here to add that all up right now, so let's just groan a little and say I've probably taken in about three days' worth of carbo-cals.

Do you want to plunge into Friday?

It starts with breakfast at beautiful Cypress Gardens and you better try a little honey on that bran muffin, sir. Lunch is two greasy cheeseburgers on the run. Dinner is on the five o'clock plane to Dallas. It starts with the creamed sea food appetizer surrounded by a sea wall of mashed potatoes. Then it's pork chops lying in thickened gravy, candied sweet potatoes, apple sauce and peas and then the tiniest piece of pineapple cheesecake. Despite these knockout punches aimed at my dieting, I *did* make one valiant try. I declined the second roll and butter.

We arrived in Dallas and I was greeted by a large sign that read "The _____ Hotel Welcomes Ed McMahon." Upstairs the welcome was in full swing. Well, sir, the welcome ended about 2 A.M., just after I wrapped my intake up with a corned beef on rye.

I'm up at 5:30 A.M. and breakfast is two cheese Danish at the Budweiser shooting location fifty miles from the hotel. Somehow I manage to find a pair of matching cheeseburgers for lunch. For dinner that evening on the flight to Winterhaven I elect the beef dinner but cannot resist the cherry cheesecake.

Back at the motel in Cypress Gardens they're out of meat loaf, but they have dry roasted cashews and so do I.

It's Sunday now and I'm back making the special at Winterhaven. It's a re-run carbo-cal-wise of Friday, because I'm on a plane back to New York for a business meeting. The late night flight has those funny sandwiches and a Hogie seeks me out.

Monday in New York I try to buckle down—scrambled eggs and bacon for breakfast but no toast or muffin. Lunch is a sirloin and salad. Getting back in the groove, but the airline does me in again. As I head back to Winterhaven via Atlanta I follow the same script, martinis, almonds, roasted peanuts, and another Hogie for my collection.

Tuesday in Cypress Gardens is another devastating one. There's honey on the muffins, cheese on the burgers and pounds on your floundering hero. Dinner that night is at Christos with all the goodies.

On the early Wednesday morning breakfast flight to New York would you believe French toast and sausage? But at least I'm fighting back by refusing the roll. Lunch is a steak, but I'm feeling sorry for myself for some reason (probably because I didn't take the roll at breakfast) and I find a breadstick or two. And butter.

Wednesday night and I'm home. Finally. After dinner I rise and in a loud, clear voice announce that I am starting the strictest diet known to man—tomorrow.

Well, naturally I don't go to that extreme, but I did manage to right my wrongs and get back on the low carbohydrate trail.

So you see what happens to me. Have a good week and five pounds are gone. Then comes the bad week. I didn't weigh myself when I returned, but I know I put those five pounds back on. I don't know how many pounds I've taken off and put back on during the past year ,or so, quite a few I imagine. But I do know one thing—I've taken off a net of thirty-two pounds during that time, thirty-two pounds in my personal fight for slimness. My eating program, despite the occasional falling-away brought on by the festive affairs and culinary delights that are made available, has been successful for me. I'm sure it can be just as successful for you. If I can do it surviving the breadstick conspiracy, the potato plot and all the other obstacles thrown in my way, then you can do it too.

I expect very shortly to attain my goal—200 pounds. And, more important, live in that neighborhood permanently.

Well, we've come a long way together. I see that it's nearly time for the make-up man to come in and start prettying me up for the show again, so I'd like to leave you with a few thoughts about losing weight and keeping it off.

I'm not going to drop ten commandments on you because that's been done and I'm not one to lift material. But let me lay a couple of thoughts on you which can help you as they are helping me.

1. Remember it's 250 carbo-cals a day. I'm not saying you stay exactly at 250 a day, but keep hovering around the figure and you'll be surprising yourself with a big start toward your new slimness in less than a week.

2. Your willpower *will* be tested, particularly at first. If you've spent thirty years doing things your way while the weight piles up, you can't change overnight without some withdrawal symptoms. Get by the first few weeks and you'll find the pressure reduced greatly because you'll *like* what you're eating and drinking and as an added incentive, you'll *like* the way you feel and the way you look.

3. Get to know which foods are high in carbo-cals. I've got carbo-caloric charts on just about every available food and drink placed at the back of the book for your reference. Don't drive yourself wild figuring it right down to the last mouthful and fraction of a calorie. That takes the fun out of one of our daily delights, eating. After a while you'll get to know the "go ahead" foods, the "hey, watch it," items and the "back off, buddy," category.

4. Don't be discouraged. There may come a time, particularly at that third week plateau, when you feel you've been going great and no weight loss is registered. Don't give up. Stay with it. It'll work.

5. Don't hate yourself in the morning when you fail. It's bound to happen. I refer with no special pride to my traveling week which I detailed earlier. Rather, let it inspire you to greater strength to get back to the winning trail.

6. Plan menus using the wide-range of tastes offered by the low carbo-cal method. At the end of the book I have some goodies for you. I've tried all of these dishes and they will please. Remember, it's the side orders that can lift a man out of the healthful, tasty, low-carbo-cal department into the "here we go again" category.

7. Don't go on fad diets such as one offering nothing but fricasseed kangaroo seven times a day. One man ate nothing but eggs every day for three months and ended up crowing "Lookie, Lookie, Lookie Here Comes Cookie" on the "Ted Mack Show." Balanced diet, solid, regular meals is the way to do it. Avoid long fasts. In the long run they can be harmful to you.

8. Exercise more. Walk when you can instead of riding.

9. Get a scale. Use it daily.

10. Think the thin man's thoughts.

Well, that seems to cover everything. I sincerely hope this works for you, that you find it a comfortable, pleasant, enjoyable way to spend your eating and drinking time while you lose weight. I *know* if you stick to it, it will take off pounds and make you feel younger. But I also like to feel that you're enjoying life as your weight moves back into that "recommended" weight department.

Oh, here comes the makeup man. Hey, I'll tell you what. If my plan works for you, let me know when you see me on the street or in the studio someday by calling out "Hey, Slim." And I'll do the same for you. Agreed?

Meanwhile eat (watch those carbo-cals), drink (same advice) and be merry . . . (live joyously) and may your every day be touched by the hand of good fortune.

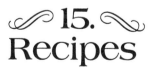

15.
Recipes

Through the years I've picked up a number of recipes from various sources during my travels and I'm listing an even dozen of them here in the hope that you'll enjoy them as much as I have.

Caesar Salad

Salt

1 clove garlic

4 small heads romaine lettuce

8 tablespoons olive oil

4 tablespoons lemon juice

4 tablespoons beer

1 one-minute coddled egg

¼ teaspoon pepper

1 cup garlic croutons

1 strip anchovy, chopped

8 tablespoons grated
   Parmesan cheese

Grated nutmeg

Sprinkle salad bowl with a little salt. Rub bowl with garlic clove. Tear lettuce leaves into thirds and place in bowl. Add olive oil, lemon juice and beer. Toss lightly until thoroughly coated. Add egg and pepper. Toss again. Add croutons, anchovy, cheese and a dash of nutmeg and toss again. Serves 8 to 10.

Shrimp Duck/USA

16 ounces beer
2 small sliced onions
1 bay leaf
3 to 4 whole peppercorns

2 whole stalks celery
1½ tablespoons salt
2 pounds shrimp, well
   washed
½ lemon, quartered

In a large pot, heat beer, onions, bay leaf, peppercorns, celery and salt. Add shrimp and lemon and simmer for 12 minutes. Allow to cool in beer. Drain and shell shrimp. Chill well. Serve with a dunking bowl of ice cold beer.

Anchovy Hash

8 hardboiled eggs
8 anchovies

2 onions
3 tablespoons butter

Mince eggs. Clean and bone anchovies, and cut them into quarter-inch pieces. Mince onions and sauté slowly, without browning, in butter. When golden, add eggs and anchovies. Heat and serve, garnished with parsley.

Barbecued Swiss Steak

2 pounds round or chuck
   steak, one-inch thick
2 eight-ounce cans seasoned
   tomato sauce
1 tablespoon each of sugar,
   vinegar, Worcestershire
   sauce

1 sliced medium onion
1/3 cup flour
salt and pepper
hot pepper sauce

Combine one-third cup flour, teaspoon of salt and half teaspoon pepper; coat meat with mixture. Brown slowly in hot fat. Pour off excess fat. Add the above spices, along with a dash or two of hot pepper sauce. Simmer uncovered for five minutes. Add onion. Cover and bake at 350 degrees for 75 minutes. Serves six.

Plain Basic Great Stew

3 pounds boneless beef
   shoulder or chuck in
   1½ inch cubes
2½ tablespoons each of
   butter and cooking oil
5 tablespoons flour
2½ teaspoons salt
5 chopped garlic cloves
1¼ teaspoons thyme
5 tablespoons finely chopped
   parsley

5 bay leaves
3 cups dry red wine
3 cups beef broth
4 medium carrots sliced
   diagonally
7 medium onions cut in
   wedges
5 halved medium potatoes
1½ teaspoons salt
¼ teaspoon pepper
1 package frozen peas

Preheat oven to 325 degrees. Be sure meat is dry. Heat butter and oil in heavy skillet and brown beef pieces slowly a few at a time. As they brown, remove them to heavy, lidded casserole with low flame under it. Sprinkle flour on meat in casserole and stir with wooden spoon until flour is absorbed. Mash garlic with salt on a saucer and add to casserole with other seasonings.

Add wine and simmer stew for five minutes. Add beef broth to cover. Place covered casserole in oven. Turn temperature down to maintain simmer.

Cook 1½ to 2 hours until beef begins to tender. Add hot water to bring it back to original level. Add vegetables, season to taste. Cover and cook 1 more hour or until meat and vegetables are tender. Tip pot, skim off fat. Add peas and cook until peas are done. Sprinkle parsley over all. Serves six.

My Type of Meat Loaf

1½ pounds ground beef
½ cup medium cracker
  crumbs
2 beaten eggs
1 cup tomato sauce

½ cup chopped green onion
3 tablespoons chopped
  green pepper
1 teaspoon salt, a pinch of
  thyme, marjoram and
  chili sauce

Put all ingredients together except chili sauce. Mix well. Form a loaf-shape and place in baking dish. Score loaf by pressing top with wooden spoonhandle, fill spaces with chili sauce. Bake one hour and 15 minutes at 350 degrees. Serves six to eight.

Cheese Omelet

6 eggs
3 tablespoons butter

¼ cup milk
3 slices American cheese
  torn into strips

Melt butter in large frying pan while preparing eggs. Break eggs in bowl, add milk and salt and pepper to taste. Beat lightly with eggbeater or fork, then pour into hot melted butter. Cover pan and cook over low heat until eggs are creamy and lightly cooked. Place cheese on one half of omelet. Fold rest of omelet over cheese, using spatula. Cook one minute.

Ranch Ribs

4 pounds loin ribs or
  spareribs sawed in
  two strips
1 cup catsup
1 tablespoon each of
  Worcestershire sauce,
  sugar, salt, celery
  seed

1 cup water
¼ cup vinegar
2 dashes hot pepper
  sauce

Season ribs with salt and pepper, then place in roasting pan. Roast for half hour at 450 degrees. Lower temperature to 350 degrees; let roast another 30 minutes. Spoon off excess fat. Combine remaining ingredients; bring to boil and pour over ribs. Continue roasting at 350 degrees for 45 minutes or until ribs are done, basting with sauce every 15 minutes. Add water if needed. Serves four.

Chicken with Pimiento Olives
(try this on your table skillet)

2½ to 3-pound ready-to-
  cook frying chicken
½ cup flour
1 teaspoon salt
¼ teaspoon pepper
¼ cup shortening

10½-ounce can cream of
  mushroom soup
1 cup water
1 small onion, sliced
¼ cup sliced pimiento
  olives

Cut chicken into quarters, half white, half dark. Mix flour, salt and pepper in paper bag. Shake chicken in flour mixture to coat evenly. Melt shortening in a skillet. Add chicken and brown it well. Heat soup and water together and pour over chicken. Spread sliced onion over top. Cover and bake for 1 hour at 350 degrees. Remove cover and stir in a little milk if needed to make one cup of gravy. Cover chicken with olives. Cover. Bake 10 minutes. Serves four.

Sweet-Sour Pot Roast

5 pounds beef pot roast   1 cup vinegar
1½ tablespoons fat   ½ cup brown sugar
½ cup sliced onion   ¼ teaspoon nutmeg

Brown roast in hot fat in kettle. Add onions. Cook until you can see through them. Add vinegar, sugar, nutmeg. Cover tightly and simmer 3½ hours or until easily penetrated with a fork. Add whatever vegetables (the low carbohydrate type, of course) you please. Serves eight.

Hash
(King of the Leftovers)

1 cup ground cooked beef   1 teaspoon salt
1 cup ground cooked   2 teaspoons Worcestershire
  potatoes   sauce
¼ cup each chopped   2/3 cup evaporated milk
  parsley and ground   ¼ cup bread crumbs
  onion   1 tablespoon melted butter

Mix beef, potatoes, onion, parsley, salt, pepper, Worcestershire sauce and milk. Place into greased one-quart casserole. Mix bread crumbs and butter. Sprinkle over top. Bake at 350 degrees for 30 minutes. Serves four.

Chinese Shrimp (Cantonese)

2 dozen shrimp (cooked,   4 ounces soy sauce
  shelled, deveined)   4 ounces lemon juice
1 bunch water cress   1 teaspoon ginger

Chill shrimp until ready to serve. Place shrimp on serving dish, garnish with water cress sprigs. Mix soy sauce, lemon juice and ginger. Divide mixture evenly into four individual serving dishes as dip for shrimp and water cress.

Lamb Kabobs

1½ pounds shoulder of lamb   ½ pound button mushrooms
½ cup French dressing   4 slices bacon
1 clove garlic   1 teaspoon salt
                                ¼ teaspoon pepper

Cut lamb into one-inch cubes. Pour French dressing over lamb, adding garlic if dressing contains none. Let stand an hour or more. Wash mushroom caps. Cut bacon into one-inch pieces. Alternate lamb, bacon, and mushrooms on metal skewers, allowing space between for thorough cooking. Season with salt and pepper. Broil three inches from heat source for 15 minutes. Turn to brown evenly. Serves six.

Salad Crab Louie

2 cups fresh or canned   ½ cup chopped fresh
  crab meat   tomato
2 tablespoons lemon   1 small chopped onion
  juice   ½ cup mayonnaise
3 cups lettuce,   2 hard-cooked eggs,
  shredded   sliced
½ cup chopped celery   1 pimiento, cut in
                                  strips

Place crab meat in bowl and sprinkle with lemon juice, tossing lightly with fork. Add lettuce, tomato, celery, onion and mayonnaise. Again use fork to toss. Place on lettuce leaf and garnish with egg slices and pimiento strips. Serves six.

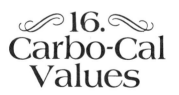

16.
Carbo-Cal
Values

Chart Contents

Key to Symbols
O few carbo-cals
□ caution required
+ heavy in carbo-cals

From the book *Martinis & Whipped Cream* by Sidney Petrie and Robert B. Stone © 1966 by Parker Publishing Company, Inc. Published by Parker Publishing Co., Inc., West Nyack, New York.

ALCOHOLIC BEVERAGES

ITEM	PORTION	CARBO-CALS	CALORIES
Ale +			
Domestic +	8 oz. beer	32	150
Imported +	8 oz. beer	40	160
Alexander, Brandy □	3 oz. cocktail	12	185
Alexander, Gin □	3 oz. cocktail	12	180
Anisette +	1 oz. cordial	28	80
Apple Jack O	1 oz. pony	2	100
Bacardi Cocktail □	3 oz. cocktail	14	100
B & B □	1 oz. pony	7	80
Beer, Bock +	8 oz. beer	35	175
Beer, Half and Half +	8 oz. beer	30	135
Beer, Lager +	8 oz. beer	30	125
Benedictine +	1 oz. cordial	26	80
Bloody Mary □	6 oz.	20	150
Bourbon & Soda			
(Highball) O	8 oz.	0	100
Bourbon & Ginger			
(Highball) +	8 oz.	65	250
Bourbon O	1½ oz.	0	100
Brandy, Apricot O	1 oz. cordial	0	75
Brandy, California O	1 oz. cordial	0	70
Brandy Cocktail O	3 oz. cordial	0	70
Brandy, Imported O	1 oz. cordial	0	75
Brandy Sour +	6 oz. delmonico	24	155
Brandy Toddy +	6 oz. old fashioned	20	140
Bronx Cocktail □	3 oz. cordial	15	105
Buttered Rum			
(Hot Toddy) O	8 oz. T & J Mug	0	350
Canadian Whiskey O	1 oz. pony	0	100
	1½oz.	0	150
Chablis O	4 oz. wine	2	140
Champagne			
domestic □	4 oz.	12	100
French O	4 oz.	4	80
Champagne Cocktail +	4 oz.	36	175
Chartreuse +	1 oz. cordial	26	85
Cherry Heering +	1 oz. cordial	24	100
Cider (Fermented) □	6 oz.	7	50
Claret Wine O	4 oz. wine	2	125

ITEM	PORTION	CARBO-CALS	CALORIES
Cognac ○	1 oz. pony	0	75
Creme de Cocoa +	1 oz. cordial	24	95
Creme de Menthe +	1 oz. cocktail	24	90
Creme de Menthe			
Frappe +	3 oz. cocktail	28	120
Cuba Libre +	10 oz. Tom Collins	40	205
Curacao +	1 oz.	24	100
Daiquiri +	3 oz. cocktail	20	180
Dubonnet +	3 oz. cocktail	48	155
French '75 +	8 oz. highball	38	280
Gin ○	1½ oz. jigger	0	112
	1 oz. pony	0	75
Gin Buck +	10 oz. highball	30	165
Gin Collins +	10 oz. Tom Collins	24	155
Gin Fizz +	10 oz. highball	28	165
Gin Rickey □	10 oz. highball	6	140
Grasshopper +	3 oz. cocktail	72	235
Horse's Neck +	10 oz. Tom Collins	36	190
Irish Coffee +	6 oz.	22	80
Irish Whiskey ○	1 oz. pony	0	100
	1½ oz.	0	150
Jack Rose +	3 oz. cocktail	18	145
Kummel +	3 oz. cocktail	24	80
Madeira +	3½ oz.	18	120
Manhattan +	3 oz. cocktail	32	260
Martini (Dry) ○	3 oz. cocktail	1	200
Martini (Sweet) +	3 oz. cocktail	32	190
Mint Julep □	10 oz. Tom Collins	12	355
Muscatel +	3½ oz.	56	170
Old Fashioned +	3 oz.	30	175
Orange Blossom +	3 oz. cocktail	16	165
Pink Lady □	3 oz. cocktail	12	170
Planter's Punch +	10 oz. Tom Collins	32	365
Port +	4 oz. wine	68	135
	3½ oz.	56	110
Porter or Stout +	8 oz.	40	200
Riesling □	4 oz. wine	8	135
Rhine Wine □	4 oz. wine	8	150
Rob Roy			
w/dry vermouth ○	3 oz. cocktail	1	110
regular +		32	230

ITEM	PORTION	CARBO-CALS	CALORIES
Rum Collins +	10 oz. Tom Collins	36	175
Rum Fizz +	8 oz. highball	28	125
Rum & Cola +	8 oz. highball	80	260
Rum Jamaica O	1 oz. pony	0	100
Rum Bacardi O	1 oz. pony	0	60
Rum Punch +	8 oz. punch cup	32	300
Rye Highball			
w/soda O	8 oz. highball	0	100
w/ginger ale +		64	200
Rye Whiskey O	1 oz. pony	0	100
	1½ oz.	0	150
Sauterne (sweet) +	4 oz. wine	20	95
	3½ oz.	16	80
Sazerac □	3 oz. cocktail	10	180
Scotch Manhattan +	6 oz. old fashioned	0	85
Scotch Mist O	3 oz. cocktail	32	235
Scotch & Soda O	8 oz. highball	0	90
Scotch Whiskey O	1 oz. pony	0	85
	1½ oz.	0	130
Screwdriver +	8 oz.	60	250
Sherry +	2½ oz. sherry	14	95
	3½ oz.	20	130
Sidecar +	3 oz. cocktail	18	150
Singapore Sling +	8 oz. highball	60	175
Sloe Gin O	1 oz. pony	0	55
	1½ oz. jigger	0	85
Sloe Gin Collins +	10 oz. Tom Collins	30	170
Sloe Gin Fizz +	8 oz. highball	15	155
Sloe Gin Rickey +	10 oz. highball	25	150
Stinger +	3 oz. cocktail	36	185
Stout +	8 oz. beer	50	140
Tom Collins +	10 oz. Tom Collins	36	155
Tom & Jerry +	8 oz. T & J mug	60	335
Vermouth (Dry or French) O	4 oz. wine	5	105
	3½ oz.	4	92
Vermouth (Sweet or Italian) +	4 oz. wine	55	175
	3½ oz.	48	153
Vodka O	1½ oz. jigger	0	180
Ward Eight +	8 oz. stem	30	230

ITEM	PORTION	CARBO-CALS	CALORIES
Whiskey Fizz +	8 oz. highball	20	160
Whiskey Highball (Soda) ○	8 oz. highball	0	175
Whiskey Sour +	3 oz. cocktail	16	200
Wine, Dry Red ○ (Chianti, Claret, Burgundy)	3½ oz.	2	70
Wine, Sour ○	3½ oz. (Dry)	2	95
Wine, Sweet +	4 oz. wine	40	130
Wine, Dry White ○ (Chablis, Moselle, Rhine)	3½ oz.	2	75
Zinfandel □	4 oz. wine	10	85
Zombie +	14 oz.	100	500

BEVERAGES

ITEM	PORTION	CARBO-CALS	CALORIES
Apple Juice +	1 cup canned	120	124
	1 cup fresh	120	123
Apricot Juice, +	1 cup	120	175
unsweetened	4 oz. glass	60	80
Apricot Nectar +	1 cup	144	160
Blackberry Juice +	1 cup	80	70
	4 oz. glass	40	35
Blueberry Juice +	4 oz. glass	56	130
Carbonated Soda +			
(Sweet)	8 oz.	80	105
Carbonated Water,			
Seltzer O	8 oz.	0	5
Carrot Juice +	1 cup	50	50
	4 oz. glass	25	25
Cherry Soda +	8 oz.	80	80
Chocolate Beverage +			
(w/milk)	1 cup	68	140
Cider, Apple			
(sweet) +	8 oz.	100	115
Clam Juice □	4 oz. glass	8	45
Cocoanut Milk □	8 oz. glass	8	60
Coffee O	8 oz.	0	0
Cola Type			
Beverages +	8 oz.	100	105
Cranberry Juice +	1 cup	140	140
Cream Soda +	8 oz.	100	105
Currant Juice +			
Black	1 cup	136	140
Red	1 cup	100	110
Egg & Fruit Punch +	8 oz.	110	275
Eggnog +	8 oz.	100	270
(All milk & one egg)			
Fruit Punch +	8 oz. glass	170	200
Ginger Ale			
(Pale Ale) +	8 oz.	84	100
Grapefruit Juice +	1 cup	82	87
canned, unsweetened +	1 cup	90	92
canned, sweetened +	1 cup	120	131
frozen, unsweetened +	6 oz. can	288	297

ITEM	PORTION	CARBO-CALS	CALORIES
frozen, unsweetened, diluted +	1 cup	96	105
frozen, sweetened +	6 oz. can	320	340
frozen, sweetened, diluted +	1 cup	112	125
Grape Juice +	1 cup	172	180
frozen, sweet +	1 cup	128	130
undiluted +	4 oz. glass	80	85
Grape Soda +	8 oz.	90	100
Grapefruit-Orange +			
canned, sweetened +	8 oz. glass	125	131
canned, sweetened +	3 fl. oz.	48	52
canned, unsweetened +	8 oz. glass	90	99
canned, unsweetened □	3 fl. oz.	35	40
frozen, condensed +	1 can–6 fl. oz.	280	297
frozen, condensed, diluted 1–3 □	3 fl. oz.	38	42
frozen, condensed, undiluted □	3 fl. oz.	130	149
Kaffee Hag ○	8 oz.	0	0
Lemonade, diluted +	1 cup	112	120
canned +	4 oz.	60	60
Pepsi Cola +	8 oz.	108	120
Pineapple Juice-Ade +	8 oz.	90	95
Pineapple Juice, canned +	½ cup	60	60
frozen, sweetened +	½ cup	60	97
Pomegranate Juice +	4 oz.	60	75
Postum, black ○	8 oz.	0	0
Prune Juice, canned +	4 oz.	80	85
Quinine Water □	8 oz.	36	40
Raspberry Juice +	4 oz.	60	66
Root Beer +	8 oz.	98	100
Sarsaparilla +	8 oz.	98	100
Sauerkraut Juice □	4 oz.	16	25
Seltzer, See Carbonated Water			
Tangerine Juice, Canned +	1 cup	108	110
canned, unsweetened +	1 cup	100	110
frozen, diluted +	1 cup	108	120
frozen, undiluted +	6 oz. can	320	330
fresh +	4 oz.	40	48

ITEM	PORTION	CARBO-CALS	CALORIES
Tea ○	8 oz.	0	0
w/lemon ○	8 oz.	1	2
See Chart for Milk & Sugar			
Tomato Juice □	1 cup	40	50
	4 oz.	20	25
Vegetable Juice □	1 cup	36	50
	4 oz.	18	25
V-8 Juice □	1 cup	36	50
	4 oz.	18	25

BREADS

ITEM	PORTION	CARBO-CALS	CALORIES
Bagel +	1 med. size	120	125
Baking Powder Biscuits +	2½" diameter	80	130
	1 small	56	90
Banana Bread +	1 slice	88	100
Blueberry Muffin +	2½" diameter	92	100
Boston Brown Bread +	slice ¾"	84	86
Unenriched flour +	slice	90	105
Degermed flour +	slice	86	100
Bran Bread +	slice	68	75
w/raisins +	slice	108	120
Bran Muffins +	3½" diameter	80	85
Bread Crumbs, dry +	½ cup	120	170
Brown Nut Bread +	slice	96	100
Cinnamon Buns +	2½" sq.	100	140
w/raisins +	1	112	155
Cinnamon Bread +	1 slice	94	135
Cinnamon Toast +	1 slice	90	130
Clover Leaf Roll +	1	80	150
Corn Muffins +	1	72	105
Cornmeal Muffins +	2¾" diameter	80	135
Corn Bread +	1 qu. pc.	70	105
Date Muffins +	2¾" diameter	130	140
Date & Nut +	slice	102	105
Egg Muffins +	2½" diameter	80	85
English Muffin, toasted +	1	120	125
Frankfurter Roll +	1	40	160
French Bread +	1 sm. slice	42	70
French Roll, Hard +	3½" diameter	65	100
French Toast Without syrup +	1 pc.	56	130
w/1 tbs. corn syrup +	1 pc.	120	250
w/1 tbs. maple syrup +	1 pc.	125	260
Gingerbread +	1 square	40	180
Gluten Bread +	slice	32	35
Graham +	slice	44	75
Hamburger Roll +	1 reg.	80	155

ITEM	PORTION	CARBO-CALS	CALORIES
Hard Roll +	1	100	155
Hot Cross Bun +	1	80	180
Italian +	1 sm. slice	40	50
Melba Toast +	slice	32	40
Pecan Buns +	1	108	150
Petit Fours +	1	100	180
Plain Muffins +	2¾" diameter	64	135
Onion Roll +	4" diameter	120	150
Parkerhouse Roll +	1	75	125
Plain Biscuits or Buns +	1	80	125
w/enriched flour +	1	85	135
Popover +	1	10	60
Protein +	slice	36	60
Pumpernickel +	slice	60	75
Raisin +	slice	70	80
Raisin Muffins +	1 regular	108	130
Roman Meal +	1 slice	52	80
Rye +			
light +	1 slice	60	75
dark +	1 slice	56	70
Party Sliced +	1 slice	32	40
Rye & Wheat +	1 slice	56	70
Soya +	1 slice	35	65
Soy Muffins +	1 medium	64	80
Spoon Bread +	1 serving	68	110
Swedish Health Bread +	2" square	30	50
Sweet Rolls +	3½" diameter	84	135
Vienna +	1 sm. slice	40	55
White, slice +	1 slice	48	64
White, plain Muffin +	1 medium	68	135
Cracked Wheat +	slice	48	80
Whole Wheat +	slice	44	55
Whole Wheat Muffin +	1 medium	68	130
Whole Wheat Roll +	1 medium	68	90
Zweiback +	1 pc.	20	25

CEREALS

ITEM	PORTION	CARBO-CALS	CALORIES
All Bran +	8 oz. cup	168	180
	½ cup	84	90
Barley +	1 tbs.	40	50
Bran Flakes,			
40% Bran +	8 oz. cup	100	115
Bran, Raisin +	8 oz. cup	120	149
Bran, Whole Cereal +	8 oz. cup	40	240
Cheerios +	8 oz. cup	68	98
Corn Flakes +	8 oz. cup	84	95
Cream of Wheat,			
cooked +	8 oz. cup	100	110
Farina, cooked +	8 oz. cup	52	120
Force +	8 oz. cup	60	180
Grapenuts +	8 oz. cup	320	400
Grapenuts Flakes +	¾ cup	72	220
Infants, Dry,			
precooked +	1 oz.	80	100
K Cereal +	1 serving	48	105
Kellogg's Concentrate +	½ cup	28	100
Kix Cereal +	8 oz. cup	80	128
Krispies +	8 oz. cup	120	136
Krumbles +	8 oz. cup	110	142
Maypo, Coat Cooked +	¾ cup	84	140
Oat Cereal, Ready-to-			
Eat +	8 oz. cup	68	100
Oatmeal, Infant Dry,			
precooked +	1 oz. portion	60	106
Oatmeal, Cooked +	8 oz. cup	104	148
Dry, Rolled Oats +	8 oz. cup	85	312
Pablum Cereal +	½ cup - 4 oz.	50	90
Pep Cereal +	8 oz. cup	90	125
Post Toasties +	8 oz. cup	80	110
Puffed Corn +	¾ cup	100	120
Puffed Rice +	8 oz. cup	46	55
Puffed Wheat +	8 oz. cup	40	55
Sweetened +	1 oz.	68	80
Ralston Health Cereal +	8 oz. cup	120	200
Ralston, Hot or			
Instant uncooked +	½ cup	80	95

ITEM	PORTION	CARBO-CALS	CALORIES
Ralston Wheat Chex +	½ cup	90	120
Rice Flakes +	8 oz. cup	108	120
Rice Krispies +	8 oz. cup	100	125
Rolled Oatmeal, cooked +	8 oz. cup	110	148
Rolled Oatmeal, infant, dry, precooked +	1 oz. portion	90	106
Rolled Oats, Cereal (Ready-to-Eat) +	8 oz. cup	80	100
Roman Meal +	½ cup	100	135
Rye Flakes +	8 oz. cup	75	125
Scotch Oatmeal, cooked +	8 oz. cup	118	150
Shredded Wheat, Biscuit +	1 oz. piece	72	100
Sugar Krisp +	1 cup	104	160
Wheat Flakes +	8 oz. cup	92	125
Wheat Germ +	2 tbs.	40	78
Wheat Meal, cereal +	8 oz. cup	118	175
Wheat & Malted Barley, cooked +	¾ cup	85	110
Wheatena, cooked +	2/3 cup	80	105
Wheaties, cereal +	8 oz. cup	92	125
Whole Meal, cooked +	8 oz. cup	160	175
Whole Meal, cooked w/wheat germ +	8 oz. cup	90	133

CHEESES

ITEM	PORTION	CARBO-CALS	CALORIES
American Cheese ○	1 slice/1 oz.	trace	100
Dry and grated ○	1 tbs.	trace	35
Fresh and grated ○	1 tbs.	trace	35
Blue Cheese ○	1 tbs.	trace	52
	1 oz.	trace	100
Domestic ○	1 oz.	trace	100
Brie ○	1 square pc.	trace	100
	1 oz.	trace	100
Camembert Cheese ○	1 triangle/1 oz.	trace	85
Chateau Cheese ○	1 oz. pc.	trace	100
Cheddar Cheese ○	1" cube/1 oz.	trace	113
Processed ○	1" cube/1 oz.	trace	105
Cottage Cheese □	8 oz. cup	16	240
	1 oz.	2	30
Creamed □	8 oz. cup	24	230
Cream Cheese ○	1 oz.	trace	106
	1 tbs.	trace	56
Edam Cheese ○	1 oz.	trace	120
Farmer Cheese ○	4 oz. pc.	trace	155
Gorgonzola Cheese ○	1 oz. pc.	trace	100
Grated Cheese, Dry ○	1 tbs.	trace	35
Grated Cheese, Fresh ○	1 tbs.	trace	30
Liederkranz Cheese ○	2 tbs.	trace	100
Limburger Cheese ○	2 tbs.	trace	97
Mysost +	1 oz.	60	130
Neufchatel Cheese ○	1 tbs.	trace	50
Pabst-ett ○	1 oz.	8	100
Parmesan Cheese ○	1 slice/1 oz.	trace	100
Fresh Grated ○	1 tbs.	trace	35
Dry Grated ○	1 tbs.	trace	30
Pot Cheese ○	1 tbs.	trace	25
	4 oz.	trace	55
Provolone Cheese ○	2 tbs.	trace	98
Roquefort Cheese	1" sq./1 oz.	trace	87
Cream Spread ○	2 tbs.	trace	102
Cheese Soufflé □	½ cup	20	280
Cheese Spreads □			
Bacon □	1 oz.	8	

ITEM	PORTION	CARBO-CALS	CALORIES
Old English Cheese			
Spread □	2 tbs.	8	100
Olive Pimento			
Spread □	2 tbs.	8	87
Pimento Spread □	2 tbs.	8	102
	1 oz.	8	100
Pineapple Spread □	1 oz.	8	100
Relish Spread □	1 oz.	8	100
Roka Spread □	1 oz.	8	100
Swiss Cheese,			
Processed ○	1 slice/1 oz.	trace	101
	1 slice/1 oz.	trace	105
Gruyere Cheese ○	1 slice/1 oz.	trace	98
Velveeta □	1 oz.	12	100
Welsh Rarebit +	1 slice and 4 tbs.	88	200

EGGS

ITEM	PORTION	CARBO-CALS	CALORIES
Boiled in Shell O	1 medium	trace	77
Creamed eggs □	2 eggs, 2 tbs. sauce	52	270
Deviled □	2 halves of med. egg	16	135
Dried, Whites O	8 oz. cup	trace	223
Dried, Whole O	8 oz. cup	trace	640
Dried, Yolks O	8 oz. cup	trace	666
Duck Eggs O	1 large	8	190
Fried O	1 medium	2	100
Eggs A La Goldenrod +	6 tbs.	72	170
Omelette O	1 med.	trace	106
Cheese (1 slice) O	2 eggs	4	250
Spanish w/milk □	2 eggs	30	200
Poached O	1 medium	trace	77
Poached in Jelly □	1 medium	30	100
Raw, Whole O	1 medium	trace	77
Scrambled O	1 medium	2	106
Stuffed O	2 medium halves	8	125
Timbale □	5 tbs.	12	117
Turkey Eggs O	1	10	248
White Only O	1 medium egg	trace	15
Yolk Only O	1 medium egg	trace	61

FISH

ITEM	PORTION	CARBO-CALS	CALORIES
Abalone			
Broiled ○	3½ oz.	trace	107
Canned ○	3½ oz.	trace	80
Dry ○	3½ oz.	trace	309
Raw ○	3½ oz.	trace	107
Anchovies ○	8 small fillets	trace	54
Paste ○	1 tsp.	trace	20
Bass ○			
Baked or Broiled ○	4 oz. portion	trace	180
Canned ○	4 oz. portion	trace	185
Raw ○	4 oz. portion	0	175
Bluefish ○			
Baked or Broiled ○	1 med. pc.	0	193
Baked or Broiled ○	1 pound	0	703
Fried ○	1 med. pc.	0	307
	1 pound	0	703
Butterfish ○			
Baked or Broiled ○	3 oz. portion	0	176
Catfish ○	3 oz. portion	0	168
Caviar ○	2 tbs.	4	70
Clams ○			
Canned ○	3 oz. solid & liquid	trace	44
Canned			
Cherrystone ○	4 oz. meat	16	90
Little Neck ○	4 oz. meat	16	90
Steamers ○	4 oz. meat	16	85
Raw, Meat Only ○	5 - 10	12	80
Steamed ○	6 w/butter	16	140
Stuffed, Baked □	2	40	180
Cod ○	3½ oz. portion	0	98
Codfish ○			
Balls □	2 small balls	40	75
Baked +	1 medium	60	125
Creamed +	8 oz. cup	64	160
Dry □	1 oz. portion	20	106
Raw ○	4 oz. portion	trace	84
Salted ○	3½ oz. portion	trace	130
Steak ○	1 medium pc.	0	100

ITEM	PORTION	CARBO-CALS	CALORIES
Crab			
Cracked O	1 medium size	10	95
Hard Shell O	3½ oz. portion	10	90
Soft Shell □	3½ oz. portion	32	90
Crabmeat, Cooked O			
Canned O	8 oz. meat	10	215
Deviled □	1 medium crab	40	200
Fresh O	3 oz. meat	3	90
Salad □	4 oz. portion	30	150
Crab Jambalaya +	1 serving	60	180
Crab Paste O	1 tsp.	trace	30
Croaker, Fresh O	4 oz. portion	trace	109
Croquettes, Fish +	1 medium	64	120
Eel, Fresh O	4 oz. portion	0	183
Eel, smoked O	4 oz. portion	0	185
Finnan Haddie O	4 oz. portion	0	100
Smoked O	4 oz. portion	0	100
Fish			
Creamed □	½ cup	32	100
Cakes +	1	40	80
Sticks, Frozen +	4 oz.	30	90
Flounder O	4 oz. portion	0	78
Frogs Legs O	4 oz. portion	0	75
fried O	4 oz. portion	4	170
Gefilte Fish □	4 oz. portion	40	75
Haddock O			
Cooked O	1 fillet	0	158
Cooked O	1 lb.	0	676
Creamed □	4 oz. portion	24	150
Fried □	1 fillet	32	165
Fried O	1 lb.	trace	748
Smoked O	4 oz. portion	0	132
Halibut O			
Broiled or cooked O	1 steak (med.)	0	228
Broiled or cooked O	1 lb. net	trace	827
Creamed □	4 oz. portion	24	170
Smoked O	4 oz. portion	0	150
Herring O			
Atlantic O	4 oz. portion	0	216
Kippered O	4 oz. portion	0	240
Lake O	4 oz. portion	0	160

ITEM	PORTION	CARBO-CALS	CALORIES
Pacific ○	4 oz. portion	0	105
Pickled ○	4 oz. portion	0	102
Pickled with sour cream ○	4 oz. portion	8	245
Smoked ○	4 oz. portion	0	240
Lobster ○			
Canned ○	3 oz. portion	trace	80
Canned ○	½ cup	trace	100
Creamed □	½ cup, 4 oz.	24	150
Fresh, Meat Only ○	3 oz.	trace	75
Fresh, w/2 tbs. butter ○	1	3	300
Baked or Broiled ○	1 average	3	120
Broiled ○	1 African Tail	0	150
Lobster Cantonese +	1 serving	30	200
Lobster Cocktail □	1 average	20	80
	½ cup meat, 2 tbs. sauce	32	90
	½ cup meat, wedge lemon	2	70
	½ cup meat, mayonnaise	trace	90
Lobster Newburgh □	½ cup	30	120
Lobster Paste ○	1 tsp	trace	25
Lobster Thermador □	1 lobster	56	200
Lox, Nova Scotia, Smoked ○	3 oz. portion	0	285
Mackerel ○			
Canned, Atlantic ○	3 oz. portion	0	155
Canned, Pacific ○	3 oz. portion	0	153
Fresh ○	3½ oz. portion	0	159
Salt ○	4 oz. portion	0	175
Mussels ○	6 medium size	trace	75
	1 lb.	28	250
Meskalunge ○	4 oz. portion	trace	100
Oysters			
Fried □	3 lg. pcs.	40	250
Raw, Blue Point ○	4 oz. meat	8	100
Raw, Blue Point ○	6-9 medium size	8	100

ITEM	PORTION	CARBO-CALS	CALORIES
Oysters			
Raw, Cape Cod ○	4 oz. meat	8	100
Raw, Cape Cod ○	5-8 medium size	8	100
Stewed, Creamed □	8 oz. cup	40	250
Raw □	1 cup (13-19)	32	170
Scalloped +	6	120	250
Oyster Stew			
½ cream,			
½ milk □	8 oz. cup	88	200
Perch			
Lake ○	4 oz. portion	0	75
Sea ○	4 oz. portion	0	85
Fried ○	3 oz.	trace	85
Pickerel ○			
Sauteed □	4 oz.	24	208
Pike ○			
Northern ○	4 oz. portion	0	85
Wall Eyed ○	4 oz. portion	0	87
Porgy ○	4 oz. portion	0	110
Red Fish ○	4 oz. portion	0	100
Red Snapper ○	4 oz. portion	0	95
Rock Cod ○			
Broiled ○	4 oz.	0	122
Sauteed ○	4 oz.	0	173
Salmon ○			
Baked, Broiled ○	medium portion	0	204
Chinock ○	3 oz. portion	0	173
Chum ○	3 oz. portion	0	140
Cohoe ○	3 oz. portion	0	140
Creamed □	½ cup-4 oz.	64	200
Humpback ○	3 oz. portion	0	122
King ○	3 oz. portion	0	173
Shrimps			
Canned-Drained ○	3 oz. portion	trace	110
Canned-solids &			
liquids ○	3 oz. portion	0	76
Fresh ○	6 medium	trace	75
Fried □	6 medium-3½ oz.	32	100
Shrimp Scampi □	6 in garlic butter	trace	175
Shrimp Cocktail □	1/3 cup w/sauce	40	80
Shrimp Creole +	6 shrimp w/sauce	100	160

ITEM	PORTION	CARBO-CALS	CALORIES
Smelts ○	2 small size	0	50
Fried w/butter +	2-3	40	150
Snails ○	6 medium size	trace	52
Sole ○			
Fillet of ○	4 oz. portion	0	100
Sauteed ○	4 oz. portion	4	236
Squid, Raw ○	3½ oz. portion	0	78
Dried ○	3½ oz. portion	0	305
Sturgeon, Smoked ○	2½ oz. portion	0	100
Swordfish ○	1 pc.	0	223
Trout ○			
Brook ○	3½ oz. portion	0	50
Brook, smoked ○	3 oz. portion	0	100
Lake ○	3 oz. portion	0	60
Lake, smoked ○	3 oz. portion	0	110
Tuna ○			
Canned, Drained ○	3 oz. portion	0	170
Canned, w/oil			
(Wet Pack) ○	3 oz. portion	0	247
Creamed ○	½ cup - 4 oz.	8	270
Fresh ○	3 oz. portion	0	150
Smoked ○	2½ oz. portion	0	125
Tuna Casserole			
w/noodles +	1 average portion	100	300
Turtle ○	½ cup - 4 oz.	0	160
Whale Meat ○	3½ oz. portion	0	116
Whitefish ○			
Broiled ○	4 oz. portion	0	125
Fried ○	4 oz. portion	0	200
Baked, Stuffed ☐	1 serving	44	260

FRUIT

ITEM	PORTION	CARBO-CALS	CALORIES
Apple +	1 large	100	160
Apple +	1 medium	64	85
Apple +	1 small	44	60
Baked w/sugar +	1 medium	150	200
Baked w/sugar +	1 large	200	260
Dried, Cooked, unsweetened +	¼ cup	92	102
Dried, Cooked, sweetened +	¼ cup	100	160
Applesauce +			
Canned, Infant +	1 oz. strained	20	25
Sweetened +	8 oz. cup	200	260
Unsweetened +	8 oz. cup	104	120
Apricots □			
Canned, Infant □	1 oz. strained	40	17
Canned, Syrup Pack +	4 med. size halves	80	97
Canned, Syrup Pack +	8 oz. cup halves	200	205
Canned, Water Pack □	8 oz. cup halves	80	77
Dried +	8 oz. cup halves	360	423
Dried, Cooked +	½ cup sweetened	200	220
Dried, Cooked +	½ cup unsweetened	120	130
Fresh □	3 medium size	40	54
Stewed +	8 oz. cup	360	400
Avocado, California □	½ pear	24	279
Avocado, California □	8 oz. cup of cubes	36	372
Avocado, Florida +	½ pear	44	279
Avocado, Florida +	8 oz. cup of cubes	52	372
Bananas +	1 large	115	120
Bananas +	1 medium	100	110
Diced +	1 cup	125	136
Fried +	1 medium	130	140
Sliced +	1 cup	140	150
Fritter +		44	80
Blackberries □	1 cup	72	82
Canned, Syrup Pack +	8 oz. cup	180	216

ITEM	PORTION	CARBO-CALS	CALORIES
Water Pack ☐	8 oz. cup	88	104
Low Calorie,			
Canned ☐	1 cup	72	80
Blueberries ☐	1 cup	80	85
Canned,			
Syrup Pack +	8 oz. cup	240	245
Water Pack ☐	8 oz. cup	80	90
Frozen,			
Unsweetened ☐	3 oz.	40	52
Frozen,			
Sweetened +	1 cup	150	160
Canned,			
Low Calorie ☐	1 cup	68	80
Boysenberries ☐			
Frozen,			
Sweetened +	1 cup	140	160
Frozen,			
Unsweetened ☐	1 cup	44	70
Cantaloupe ☐	½ of medium size	32	37
	1 cup diced	22	30
Casaba Melon ☐	1 wedge	40	52
Canned,			
Low Calorie ☐	2/3 cup	28	35
Gooseberries ☐	8 oz. cup	50	59
Grandilla (Passion			
Fruit) ☐	3½ oz. pulp & seeds	85	100
Grapes +			
Concord +	4 oz.	60	80
Delaware +	4 oz.	60	80
Flame Tokay +	8 oz. cup	128	150
Malaga +	8 oz. cup	128	150
Muscat +	8 oz. cup	128	150
Niagara +	1 bunch	60	80
Sultana +	8 oz. cup	128	150
Thompson Seedless +	8 oz. cup	120	140
Tokay +	8 oz. cup	128	150
Canned,			
with syrup +	1 cup	180	200
Canned,			
with water +	1 cup	88	100
Grapefruit ☐	½ large	88	104

ITEM	PORTION	CARBO-CALS	CALORIES
Grapefruit ☐	½ medium	72	75
Grapefruit ☐	½ small	45	49
Canned, Sweetened +	8 oz. cup	160	181
Canned, Unsweetened ☐	8 oz. cup	80	90
Sections ☐	8 oz. cup	70	77
Fresh Pink ☐	½ medium	65	75
Guavas ☐	1 medium	40	49
Honeydew Melon ☐	1 medium wedge	45	49
Huckleberries ☐	8 oz. cup	80	85
Kumquat ☐	3½ oz. piece	68	75
Kumquat ☐	1 tbs.	20	25
Kumquat ☐	5-6	40	45
Lemon ☐	1 medium	32	40
Lime ☐	1-2	24	26
Loganberries ☐	2/3 cup	60	70
Canned +	8 oz. cup	100	104
Dried +	3½ oz. portion	270	286
Loquat ☐	6-8	40	48
Lotus Seeds +	3½ oz. portion	300	350
Pineapple ☐			
Canned, Syrup Pack +	2 small slices	90	95
Canned, Syrup Pack +	1 large slice	90	95
Fresh, Diced ☐	8 oz. cup	70	74
Fresh, Sliced ☐	1 slice medium	40	44
Frozen +	4 oz. package	112	118
Canned, Low Calorie ☐	½ cup	44	50
Candied +	1 slice	120	150
Pitanga ☐	3½ oz.	40	51
Plantain +	3½ oz.	110	119
Plums ☐	1 medium	25	29
Fresh, Halves ☐	8 oz. cup	85	94
Canned,	8 oz. cup	200	210
Low Calorie ☐	1 cup	40	50
Poka, Hawaiian ☐	1 cup	44	60
Pomegranate +	1 medium size	70	75
Prickly Pear ☐	1 medium size	20	52

ITEM	PORTION	CARBO-CALS	CALORIES
Prunes +			
Canned, Infant +	1 oz. strained	28	28
Cooked, no sugar +	8 oz. cup	160	200
Cooked, w/sugar +	8 oz. cup	300	320
Dried, small +	1	12	14
Dried +	8 oz. cup	350	375
Pummelo ☐	3½ oz. portion	40	48
Quince ☐	1 medium size	40	45
Raisins +	4	12	14
Sugar Added +	8 oz. cup	520	572
Dried +	8 oz. cup	400	429
Dried +	1 tbs.	20	26
Raspberries ☐			
Canned +	8 oz. cup	220	250
Fresh, Black ☐	8 oz. cup	84	100
Fresh, Red ☐	8 oz. cup	65	70
Frozen +	3 oz. package	95	126
Canned,			
With Water ☐	24	35	
Rhubarb ☐	8 oz. cup	16	19
Roseapple ☐	3½ oz. portion	50	56
Sapodilla ☐	3½ oz. portion	80	89
Sapote +	3½ oz. portion	110	125
Soursop ☐	3½ oz. portion	60	65
Strawberries ☐	8 oz. cup	52	54
Frozen +	3 oz. package	80	90
Fresh ☐	5 large	20	25
Tangerine ☐	1 medium size	30	35
Watermelon ☐	½ slice	40	45
	wedge, medium	85	100
Balls or Cubes ☐	½ cup	28	35

MEATS

ITEM	PORTION	CARBO-CALS	CALORIES
BEEF ○			
Canned, Infant ○	1 oz. strained	0	30
Canned, Roast Beef ○	3 oz. portion	0	189
Brains ○	2/3 cup	6	400
Brisket ○	3½ oz.	0	380
Chipped Beef ○	8 oz. cup	0	336
with cream □	½ cup	24	175
Chuck or Cooked			
Beef ○	3½ oz. without bone	0	421
Corned Beef ○			
Boiled ○	1 med. pc.	0	100
Canned, Lean ○	3 oz.	0	159
Canned, Medium			
Fat ○	3 oz.	0	182
Canned, Fat ○	3 oz.	0	221
Corned and Hash □	1 cup	80	320
Croquettes, Beef □	1 medium	36	280
Filet Mignon ○	3½ oz. portion	0	224
Flank and Cooked			
Beef ○	3½ oz. without bone	0	235
Hamburger ○	1 lb. portion	0	1654
Hamburger ○	3 oz. portion	0	316
Dried Beef ○	1 cup	0	336
Dried Beef ○	2 oz. portion	0	115
Heart, Beef ○	3 oz. portion	2	90
Lean ○	3 oz. portion	2	164
Braised ○	3 oz. portion	3	170
Kidney Beef ○	½ cup portion	4	160
Liver, cooked □	3½ oz.	24	207
Infant ○	1 oz. strained	7	30
Lung, Beef ○	4 oz. portion	4	105
Meat Balls ○	3 oz.	0	316
Meat Loaf □	1 slice, 3 oz.	44	320
Porterhouse Steak,			
Cooked ○			
with bone ○	1 lb.	0	895
without bone ○	1 lb.	0	1100
without bone ○	3½ oz.	0	242
Pot Pie +	4¼" diameter	148	450

ITEM	PORTION	CARBO-CALS	CALORIES
Pot Roast, Cooked ○	3½ oz. portion	0	298
Rib Roast, Cooked ○			
with bone ○	1 lb.	0	1050
without bone ○	1 lb.	0	1189
without bone ○	3½ oz.	0	262
Round Steak, Regular,			
Cooked ○			
without bone ○	1 lb.	0	1040
without bone ○	3½ oz.	0	229
Round Steak, Bottom,			
Cooked ○			
with bone ○	1 lb.	0	917
without bone ○	1 lb.	0	1281
without bone ○	3½ oz.	0	250
Rump, Cooked ○			
with bone ○	1 lb.	0	850
without bone ○	1 lb.	0	1067
without bone ○	3½ oz.	0	235
Sirloin, Cooked ○			
with bone ○	1 lb.	0	800
without bone ○	1 lb.	0	944
without bone ○	3½ oz.	0	200
Stew, Beef ○	1 cup	0	350
Stew, Beef and			
Vegetable +	8 oz. cup	80	252
Sweetbreads, broiled ○	½ cup	0	100
creamed □	½ cup	24	300
Swiss Steak +	3½ oz.	68	300
T Bone Steak ○	3½ oz. portion	0	247
Tenderloin Steak ○	3½ oz. portion	0	224
Tongue, Beef,			
Medium Fat ○	3 oz.	trace	174
Pickled ○	1 tbs.	trace	32
Canned ○	4 oz. portion	trace	252
Tripe ○	½ cup	0	100
Pickled ○	3½ oz.	trace	88
LAMB			
Canned, Infant ○	1 oz. strained	0	30
Curry, Lamb +	½ cup	88	400
Kidneys ○	½ cup	4	118

ITEM	PORTION	CARBO-CALS	CALORIES
Chops O			
Broiled, without			
bone O	3½ oz.	0	223
Fried, without bone O	3½ oz.	0	270
Rib Chops, Broiled O	3½ oz.	0	291
Roast Leg O			
with bone O	1 lb.	0	720
without bone O	1 lb.	0	885
without bone O	3½ oz.	0	195
Shish Kebab, Lamb O	3½ oz.	0	300
Shoulder Roast O			
without bone O	1 lb.	0	1551
without bone O	3 oz.	0	293
with bone O	1 lb.	0	1160
Sirloin Chops O	1 medium chop	0	110
Stew, Lamb O	8 oz. cup	0	300
Stew, Lamb with			
vegetables +	8 oz. cup	44	450
Chops or Roast Mutton			
thin fat O	3½ oz.	0	206
medium fat O	3½ oz.	0	317
LIVERS			
Canned, Infant O	3½ oz.	6	100
Canned, Infant O	1 oz.	trace	30
Beef Liver □	3½ oz.	24	160
Calves Liver □	3½ oz. portion	16	140
Chicken Liver			
Broiled O	3½ oz.	6	141
Raw O	3½ oz.	6	120
Sauteed □	3½ oz.	12	155
Chicken Liver,			
Chopped □	3 oz. portion	12	150
Goose Liver □	2 medium	12	150
Lamb or Sheep □	3 oz. portion	16	116
	1 slice	12	90
Liverwurst O	2 oz. slice	2	150
Pork O	1 slice	8	320
Spread, Liver O	2 tbs./1 oz.	trace	95
Steer □	3 oz. portion	16	119
PORK, HAM			
Baked O	1 medium slice	0	265

ITEM	PORTION	CARBO-CALS	CALORIES
Boiled, with bone ○	1 lb.	0	1432
Boiled, without bone ○	1 lb.	0	1818
Boiled, without bone ○	3 oz.	0	338
Boiled, Luncheon ○	2 oz.	0	172
Deviled ○	1 tbs.	4	50
Fried ○	3 oz. portion	0	342
Hocks ○	3 oz. portion	0	340
Loaf ○	3 oz. portion	0	355
Luncheon, Canned & Spiced ○	3 oz.	trace	246
Picnic, Shoulder, Fresh ○	3½ oz.	trace	246
Prosciutto ○	1½ oz.	0	170
Smoked, with bone ○	1 lb.	trace	1496
Smoked, without bone ○	1 lb.	trace	1804
Smoked, without bone ○	3 oz.	trace	339
Spiced, Fresh, Canned ○	2 oz.	trace	165
Heart, Pork ○	3 oz. portion	trace	150
Kidneys, Pork ○	½ cup	trace	129
Pigs Feet ○			
Boiled ○	4 oz.	0	185
Pickled ○	4 oz. portion	trace	230
Boston Butt ○	3½ oz. portion	trace	283
Canned, Infant Pork ○	1 oz. strained	0	36
Canned, Spiced ○	2 oz. portion	0	165
Chops ○			
with bone ○	1 lb.	0	1149
Loin, Center Cut, without bone ○	1 lb.	0	1135
Loin, Center Cut, with bone ○	3 oz. portion	0	210
without bone ○	3½ oz. portion	0	250
Carcass			
Medium Fat ○	3½ oz. portion	0	457
Thin ○	3½ oz. portion	0	376

ITEM	PORTION	CARBO-CALS	CALORIES
Leg Roast ○	3 oz. portion	0	270
Loin ○			
Roasted with bone ○	1 lb.	0	1149
Roasted without bone ○	1 lb.	0	1508
Roasted, 1 chop ○	3½ oz.	0	293
Roasted, without bone ○	3 oz. portion	0	284
Pork ○			
Salt Pork ○	3 oz. portion	0	200
Sirloin Pork ○	3½ oz. portion	0	227
Spareribs ○	3½ oz. medium	0	351
Tenderloin, Pork ○	3½ oz. portion	0	239
Tongue ○	3½ oz. portion	trace	214
POULTRY AND GAME ○			
Chicken ○			
Boiled ○	4 oz. serving	0	75
Broiled ○	½ medium size	0	210
Canned, Boned ○	3 oz.	trace	169
Creamed □	½ cup-4 oz.	20	216
Croquettes +	1 medium size	30	105
Fat ○	1 tbs.	0	100
Fried ○	5 oz.	10	204
Fried ○	1 leg	5	65
Fried □	8 oz. ½ medium	25	255
Gizzard ○	3½ oz. serving	0	116
Heart ○	3 oz. pc.	4	134
Liver, Broiled ○	3½ oz. serving	trace	141
Raw ○	3 oz. serving	trace	120
Sauteed ○	3 oz. serving	trace	155
Raw, Broilers ○	½ bird boned	0	332
Raw, Friers, Boned ○	1 breast	0	210
Raw, Roasters, Boned ○	4 oz. pc.	0	227
Raw, Stewing Hen, Boned ○	4 oz. pc.	0	342
Chicken A La King □	½ cup	24	218
Chicken Paprikash □	Small serving	20	200

ITEM	PORTION	CARBO-CALS	CALORIES
Chicken Pie +	Small Pie	80	400
Chicken TV Dinner +	1	160	500
Duck O			
Gizzard O	3½ oz. serving	0	127
Raw O	3½ oz. serving	0	326
Raw, Dried and			
Salted O	3½ oz. serving	0	413
Roasted, Boned O	4 oz. piece	0	325
Goose O			
Gizzard O	3½ oz. serving	0	139
Raw O	3½ oz. serving	0	354
Roasted, Boned O	4 oz. piece	0	315
Patê Maison □	3 oz. portion	20	200
Patê De Fois Gras O	1 tbs.	3	75
Pheasant, Roasted,			
Boned O	4 oz. piece	0	150
Quail, Broiled O	4 oz. portion	0	150
Squab, Broiled			
boned O	3½ oz. portion	0	279
Stuffing, Meat or			
Poultry +	½ cup	112	330
Turkey			
All Dark O	4 oz. serving	0	327
All White O	4 oz. serving	0	280
Gizzard O	3½ oz. serving	0	188
Raw, Medium Fat O	4 oz. piece	0	304
Roasted O	4 oz. piece	0	318
Creamed on Toast +	1 cup	52	400
Pot Pie +	1 pie	160	420
VEAL			
Canned, Infant O	1 oz. strained	0	24
Carcass O			
Thin O	3½ oz. portion	0	156
Medium Fat O	3½ oz. portion	0	190
MISC.			
Frankfurter O	1 average	4	124
Hash			
Canned,			
Corned Beef □	3 oz.	28	155
Horsemeat O	3½ oz. portion	4	218
Pastrami O	2 medium slices	0	170

ITEM	PORTION	CARBO-CALS	CALORIES
Rabbit O	3 oz. portion	0	162
Stew □	1 cup	44	560
Sausages			
Cervelat O	1 medium piece	4	50
Pork Links O	1 link	0	63
Salami □	8 oz.	12	467
Vienna Sausage O	8 oz. portion	3	488
Polish O	8 oz.	4	450
Pork Sausage O	4 oz. portion	trace	540
Head Cheese,			
Sausage O	3 oz. piece	0	70
Tongue, Canned O	3 oz.	trace	210
Venison O	4 oz. slice	0	225
Wienerschnitzel O	4 oz. slice	4	275

SALADS

ITEM	PORTION	CARBO-CALS	CALORIES
Apple Carrot ☐	½ cup	46	270
Asparagus Tips ☐	5 med. spears	14	35
Avocado ☐	½ of med. pear	35	279
Cubed ☐	½ cup	20	186
with tomato &			
cottage cheese ☐		36	220
Banana +	1 medium used	100	310
Banana and nut +	½ banana used	60	200
Banana and Orange +	½ of each	88	210
Cabbage Slaw ☐	6 tbs.	20	50
Carrot-Raisin +	3 tbs.	112	150
Chicken Salad ☐	½ cup chicken	10	230
Crab Meat ☐	½ cup packed	12	100
Dandelion Greens ☐	1 cup packed	8	100
Deviled Meat ☐	2 tbs. rounded used	trace	150
Eggs			
Deviled ☐	2 halves used	10	148
Sliced ☐	1 medium used	trace	85
Egg and Tomato ☐	½ cup of each	16	180
Endive ☐	1 cup packed	30	50
and grapefruit ☐	1 cup packed	50	65
Escarole ☐	1 cup packed	25	50
Fig, Fresh +	3 small used	85	100
Fruit Combination			
Canned +	¾ cup	90	135
Fresh +	¾ cup	80	95
Canned +	3 tbs.	120	150
Canned,			
Low Calorie ☐	2/3 cup	28	50
Herring ☐	½ cup	20	115
Lettuce ☐	4 leaves used	trace	7
and tomato ☐	1 cup heaped	20	25
with French Dressing			
Wedge ☐		28	130
Lobster ☐	3 oz. portion used	20	85
Canned ☐	3 oz. portion	25	90
Macaroni +	1 cup	200	310
Orange and Grapefruit			
with dressing ☐	½ cup	40	200

ITEM	PORTION	CARBO-CALS	CALORIES
Pineapple ☐	½ cup used	45	115
and Cheese ☐	¾ cup portion	70	218
Potato +	½ cup	52	100
Salmon ☐	3 oz. used	10	200
Sardine ☐	3 oz. used	8	200
Seafood Combination ☐	½ cup packed	8	100
Shrimp ☐	½ cup packed	5	90
Tomato and Cheese ☐	½ cup packed	12	95
and Cucumber ☐	3 oz.	11	110
stuffed ☐	1 small used	9	75
Tossed ☐	1 cup packed	10	35
with French			
Dressing ☐	1 tbs.	20	135
Tomato and			
Cucumber ☐	3 oz.	12	90
Tomato Aspic ☐	½ cup	20	100
Tuna ☐	4 tbs. used	10	110
Vegetable			
Combination ☐	½ cup	25	40
Waldorf ☐	½ cup packed	40	145

SOUPS

ITEM	PORTION	CARBO-CALS	CALORIES
Asparagus, Creamed □	8 oz. cup	64	201
Barley □	8 oz. cup	56	117
Bean, Navy +	8 oz. cup	108	200
Beef Broth □	8 oz. cup	20	70
Beef Creamed □	8 oz. cup	50	205
Beef Noodle □	1 serving	28	100
Beef with Vegetable			
and Barley □	1 serving	35	120
Bouillon, Clear O	8 oz. cup	trace	9
cube O	1	trace	2
Celery, Creamed □	8 oz. cup	52	201
Chicken			
Broth O	8 oz. cup	0	50
Creamed □	8 oz. cup	20	200
Gumbo □	8 oz. cup	50	155
Infant Food □	1 oz. strained	trace	17
and Matzoth			
Balls □	2 balls and 1 cup	60	200
Noodle □	8 oz. cup	28	100
and Rice □	8 oz. cup	18	100
Vegetable □	8 oz. cup	30	90
Chili Beef Soup +	1 serving	75	200
Clam Chowder □			
with milk □	1 serving	28	100
with tomato □	1 serving	32	120
Consomme, Clear O	8 oz. cup	0	5
Corn Chowder,			
Creamed +	8 oz. cup	70	198
Creamed Soups			
(most) □	8 oz. cup	40	180
Duck, Creamed □	8 oz. cup	40	200
Green Pea +	1 serving	90	150
with Ham +	1 serving	100	180
Gumbo Creole □	8 oz. cup	40	100
Jellied Consomme O	1 serving	0	10
Lentil +	8 oz. cup	200	600
Mock Turtle □	8 oz. cup	50	109
Mulligatawny □	8 oz. cup		165
Mushroom, Creamed □	8 oz. cup	40	195

ITEM	PORTION	CARBO-CALS	CALORIES
Noodle ☐	8 oz. cup	28	100
Onion ☐			
Creamed ☐	8 oz. cup	28	200
French ☐	8 oz. cup	35	150
Oxtail ☐	8 oz. cup	35	150
Oyster Stew ½ cream,			
½ milk +	8 oz. cup	100	200
whole milk +	8 oz. cup	120	244
skimmed milk +	8 oz. cup	140	155
Pea +	8 oz. cup	100	200
Creamed +	8 oz. cup	80	225
Pepperpot ☐	8 oz. cup	35	175
Potato +	8 oz. cup	100	185
Creamed +	8 oz. cup	75	215
Rice +	8 oz. cup	70	117
Scotch Broth ☐	8 oz. cup	36	100
Shrimp, Creamed ☐	1 serving	44	120
Spinach ☐	8 oz. cup	44	205
Split Pea +	8 oz. cup	96	210
Creamed +	8 oz. cup	100	265
Tomato, Clear +	8 oz. cup	80	75
Creamed +	8 oz. cup	80	202
Rice +	1 serving	85	210
Vegetable ☐	1 serving	50	180
Turkey Noodle ☐	1 serving	28	100
Vegetable ☐	8 oz. cup	30	82
and Lamb, Infant ◯	1 oz. strained	trace	14
and Beef ☐	8 oz. cup	50	182
Infant ☐	1 oz. strained	trace	12
Creamed ☐	8 oz. cup	40	220
Vichyssoise ☐	1 serving	48	200

VEGETABLES

ITEM	PORTION	CARBO-CALS	CALORIES
Amaranth ☐	3½ oz.	30	36
Arrowhead ☐	3½ oz. of tubers	52	106
Arrowroot +	3½ oz.	100	126
Artichoke ☐			
Hearts, canned ☐	5	32	37
French +	1	80	120
Jerusalem ☐	4 small	68	78
Bottom ☐	1	20	30
Asparagus ☐			
Stalks, Cooked ☐	6	12	22
cut spears ☐	¾ cup	14	30
Canned,			
cut spears ☐	1 cup	24	43
Canned ☐	6 spears	12	22
Frozen ☐	6 spears	12	22
cut spears ☐	1 cup	20	36
Aster Leaves ☐	3½ oz. portion	20	31
Balsampear ☐	3½ oz.	10	29
Bamboo Shoots ☐	3½ oz.	22	27
Beans			
Baked, Canned pork			
and molasses +	1 cup	200	325
Baked, Canned,			
tomato sauce +	1 cup	180	295
Green, cooked ☐	1 cup	12	27
Green, canned ☐	¾ cup	30	50
Green, canned ☐	1 cup w/liquid	24	43
Green, strained ☐	1 oz.	4	6
Kidney +	7 tbs.	64	180
Lima +	½ cup cooked	100	130
Lima, canned +	1 cup	120	176
Lima, frozen +	3½ oz.	68	130
Bean Sprouts			
Mung ☐	1 cup	16	27
Soy ☐	1 cup	20	30
Beet Greens ☐	½ cup cooked	20	39
Beets			
Raw ☐	2 medium	40	104
Cooked ☐	½ cup	44	55

ITEM	PORTION	CARBO-CALS	CALORIES
Canned ☐	½ cup	44	60
Canned, strained ☐	1 oz.	8	10
Pickled ☐	1 cup	44	56
Broccoli ☐			
Cooked ☐	1 cup	32	44
Frozen ☐	2 - 3 spears	16	20
Brussel Sprouts,			
Cooked ☐	1 cup	32	44
Burdock Root +	3½ oz. portion	60	94
Cabbage			
Shredded ☐	1 cup	20	24
Chinese ☐	1 cup	8	14
Chinese, Cooked ☐	1 cup	16	27
1 wedge ☐		8	24
Calabash ☐	3½ oz.	8	17
Carrots ☐			
Raw ☐	1	20	21
Raw, Grated ☐	1 cup	40	45
Cooked ☐	1 cup diced	36	44
Canned ☐	1 cup diced	40	44
Canned, strained ☐	1 oz.	6	7
Cauliflower ☐			
Buds ☐	1 cup	20	25
Cooked ☐	1 cup	24	30
Frozen ☐	1 cup	28	35
Cedar Leaves ☐	3½ oz.	20	45
Celeriac ☐	4 - 6 roots	32	45
	8 - 14 roots	60	90
Celery ☐	1 lg. stalk	6	7
Diced ☐	1 cup	15	18
Cooked ☐	1 cup	18	24
Fresh ☐	3 small inner stalks	6	9
Chard ☐	1 cup cooked leaves	8	47
Leaves and Stalks ☐	1 cup cooked	25	30
Chayote ☐	3½ oz.	8	28
Chives, chopped ☐	3½ oz.	8	42
Chicory ☐	5 or 6 leaves	16	18
Chrysanthemum ☐	3½ oz.	12	17
Collards ☐	1 cup	52	76
Coriander ☐	3½ oz.	80	140

ITEM	PORTION	CARBO-CALS	CALORIES
Corn +	1 ear	120	150
	1 cup kernels	115	140
Canned, w/liquid +	1 cup	160	170
Corn Fritter +	1	40	50
Cowpeas +	1 cup cooked	100	151
Cress ☐			
Garden ☐	1 lb.	60	186
Garden ☐	1 cup cooked	40	73
Water ☐	1 lb.	60	180
Water ☐	1 bunch	20	40
Water ☐	10 sprigs	1	2
Cucumber ☐	1 medium	6	12
Dandelion Greens ☐	¾ cup cooked	52	75
Egg Plant ☐	½ cup	15	52
Endive ☐	10 leaves	4	6
Escarole ☐	2 lg. leaves	4	6
Fennel ☐	1 cup	8	12
Garlic ☐	1 clove	4	5
Ginger Root ☐	3½ oz.	28	51
Hominy Grits +	½ cup cooked	52	65
Horseradish ☐	1 tbs.	10	12
Kale ☐	½ cup cooked	32	55
Kohlrabi, cooked,			
fresh +	8 oz. cup sliced	52	72
Leeks ☐	3 medium	18	42
Lentils +	¾ cup	140	315
Lettuce ☐	1 compact head	18	68
Lotus Root +	2/3 average segment	40	49
Matai, Fresh +	3½ oz.	50	78
Mint ☐	1 tsp chopped	0	8
Mushrooms ☐	4 large	3	4
canned, 1 cup with			
liquid ☐		15	28
Sauteed ☐	7 small	10	60
Fresh ☐	8 oz. cup sliced	12	20
Button ☐	3½ oz.	8	16
Mustard, Dry ☐	1 tsp.	0	10
Mustard Greens ☐	1 cup cooked	20	31
Okra ☐	¼ cup	12	19
Olives ☐			
Green ☐	10 large	4	104

ITEM	PORTION	CARBO-CALS	CALORIES
Ripe or Black ☐	10 large	8	135
Stuffed ☐	5 mammoth	7	55
Onions			
Raw ☐	1 medium	40	49
	1 tbs. chopped	3	4
Cooked ☐	1 cup	72	79
Green ☐	6 small	20	23
Scalloped ☐	½ cup	60	70
Fried ☐	½ cup	140	162
Spanish ☐	1 medium size	6	8
Creamed ☐	½ cup	80	108
Stewed ☐	½ cup	40	50
Oyster Plant ☐	½ cup cooked	28	35
Parsley ☐	1 tbs. chopped	trace	1
Parsnips +	½ cup cooked	40	47
Raw +	3½ oz.	65	78
Peas +			
Fresh, Cooked +	1 cup	80	111
Fresh, Cooked +	1 lb. in pod	144	316
Canned, with liquid +	1 cup	132	168
Canned, Drained +	1 cup	112	145
Canned, strained +	1 oz.	8	14
Frozen +	½ cup	44	
Split, cooked +	1 cup	140	
Fresh, Garden, Shelled +	3½ oz.	75	90
Peppers ☐			
Green ☐	1 medium	12	16
Green, Stuffed ☐	1 medium	48	185
Red, Hot Dried ☐	1 tbs.	36	52
Red ☐	1 medium	16	28
Cooked ☐	1 medium	12	17
Pickle			
Chow Chow ☐	4 pcs.	4	7
Cucumber, Bread & Butter ☐	4 slices	18	20
Dill ☐	1 medium	12	15
Sweet ☐	1 large	10	22
Sour ☐	1 large	12	15
Sweet Mixed Relish ☐	1 tbs.	12	14
with mustard ☐	1 tbs.	14	16

ITEM	PORTION	CARBO-CALS	CALORIES
Pimento ☐	1 medium canned	8	10
Potato Chips +	10	40	108
Potatoes			
Au Gratin +	4 oz.	48	250
Baked or Boiled +	1 medium	80	100
Canned +	3 - 4 small	75	90
Creamed +	½ cup	56	125
French Fried +	10 pcs.	80	157
Hash Brown +	1 cup	240	470
French Fried,			
frozen +	10 pcs.	60	148
Fried +	½ cup	120	239
Mashed, with milk +	½ cup	60	79
Mashed, with			
butter +	½ cup	52	120
Baked with peel +	1 medium	80	102
Baked without peel +	1 medium	70	97
Boiled, peeled +	1 medium	75	105
Boiled, peeled +	8 oz. cup	75	105
Boiled, unpeeled +	1 medium	80	181
Boiled, unpeeled +	1 lb.	150	359
Canned, drained +	3 - 4 small	80	118
Canned, drained +	1 lb.	150	378
Mashed +	1 cup	90	240
Pressure Cooked +	1 medium	75	105
Pressure Cooked +	1 cup diced	75	105
Steamed +	1 medium	75	105
Steamed +	1 cup diced	75	105
Scalloped +	½ cup	60	121
Pumpkin +	3½ oz.	28	31
Canned +	1 cup	70	76
Radishes ☐	4 small	4	7
Chinese Radishes ☐	3½ oz.	16	19
Rice			
Converted and			
Cooked +	8 oz. cup	160	204
Fried +	8 oz. cup	160	258
Pre-Cooked Dry +	8 oz. cup	180	420
Spanish +	8 oz. cup	140	300
White, Boiled +	8 oz. cup	160	201
Wild Rice +	8 oz. cup	180	240

ITEM	PORTION	CARBO-CALS	CALORIES
Romaine ☐	¼ head	3	4
Rutabaga ☐	1 cup cooked	50	60
Sauerkraut ☐	½ cup drained	20	27
Scallions ☐	4 medium	4	8
Sesame Seeds ☐	1 oz.	0	8
Shepherdspurse ☐	3½ oz.	25	39
Sorrel ☐	4 oz. cup	trace	5
Soy Beans ☐			
Fresh ☐	½ cup	trace	119
Soybean Sprouts ☐	1 cup	24	60
Snow Peas ☐	14	20	30
Spinach ☐			
Raw ☐	½ pound	24	44
Cooked ☐	1 cup	24	46
Canned ☐	1 cup	24	46
Canned, Strained ☐	1 oz.	3	5
Tomatoes ☐			
Canned ☐	8 oz. cup	9	46
Fresh ☐	1 medium	6	30
Fresh ☐	1 small	4	22
Stewed ☐	8 oz. cup	9	50
Puree, Canned ☐	1 cup	18	90
Squash			
Hubbard or Winter,			
Baked +	½ cup	44	50
Hubbard, or Winter,			
frozen +	1 cup boiled	40	45
Summer, Boiled ☐	½ cup	16	19
Summer, Canned			
Strained ☐	1 oz.	4	8
Hubbard +	½ cup	44	50
Winter, Baked or			
Mashed +	1 cup	80	97
Winter, Boiled and			
Mashed +	1 cup	80	86
String Beans, fresh ☐	6 tbs.	16	21
Succotash +			
Canned +	½ cup	60	68
Swamp Cabbage ☐	3½ oz.	15	29
Sweet Potatoes +			
Raw +	3½ oz.	100	123

ITEM	PORTION	CARBO-CALS	CALORIES
Baked +	1	140	183
Boiled +	1	160	252
Candied +	1 small	240	314
Canned +	1 cup	216	233
Boiled +	1 lb.	330	560
Turnip Tops ☐	½ cup cooked	28	49
Turnips			
Cooked ☐	½ cup	16	22
Mashed ☐	8 oz. cup	45	20
Watercress ☐	10 pcs.	1	2
Yams			
Cooked +	1 cup	180	260
Baked, peeled +	1	160	183
Boiled, peeled +	1	170	252
Candied +	1 small	220	314
Yautia ☐	½ of 4" long piece	28	75
Zucchini ☐	½ cup	16	23

Bibliography

Davis, Adelle. *Let's Eat Right to Keep Fit.* New York, Harcourt, Brace, 1954.

Deutsch, Ronald M. *The Family Guide to Better Food and Better Health.* Des Moines, Meredith Corp., 1971.

Glenn, Morton B. *How to Get Thinner Once and For All.* New York, E. P. Dutton & Co., 1965.

Field, Hazel E. *Foods in Health and Disease.* New York, Macmillan Co., 1964.

Johnson, Dr. Harry J. *East, Drink, Be Merry & Live Longer.* Garden City, Doubleday & Co., 1965.

Guthrie, Helen Andrews. *Introductory Nutrition.* St. Louis, C. V. Mosby Co., 1967.

McHenry, E. W. *Food Without Fads.* Philadelphia, J. B. Lippincott, 1960.

Mayer, Jean. *Overweight.* Englewood Cliffs, Prentice-Hall, 1968.

Morrison, Lester M. *The Low-Fat Way to Health and a Longer Life.* Englewood Cliffs, Prentice-Hall, 1958.

Petrie, Sidney, and Stone, Robert B. *Martinis & Whipped Cream.* New York, Paperback Library, 1966.

Rodahl, Kaare. *Be Fit for Life.* New York, Harper & Row, 1966.

Stillman, Dr. Irwin M., and Baker, Samm S. *The Doctor's Quick Weight Loss Diet.* Englewood Cliffs, Prentice-Hall, 1967.

Wyden, Peter. *The Overweight Society.* New York, William Morrow & Co., 1965.

Zugibe, Frederick T. *Eat, Drink and Lower Your Cholesterol.* New York, McGraw-Hill, 1963.